LET'S GET REAL ABOUT EATING

A practical guide to nutrition and health.

LAURA KOPEC, ND, MHNE, CNC

BALBOA
PRESS
A DIVISION OF HAY HOUSE

Balboa Press books may be ordered through booksellers or by contacting:

Balboa Press
A Division of Hay House
1663 Liberty Drive
Bloomington, IN 47403
www.balboapress.com
1-(877) 407-4847

Print information available on the last page.

ISBN: 978-1-4525-7427-1 (sc)
ISBN: 978-1-4525-7428-8 (e)

Balboa Press rev. date: 08/23/2016

This book is dedicated to Anthony Orchard, my husband, my friend, and my partner in all things. You gave me the support and inspiration to pursue my true passion.

TABLE OF CONTENTS

Foreword ix

Acknowledgements. xiii

A Note to the Reader xv

Introduction. xvii

Part I—Let's get real about additives, pesticides, and GMO's.

Chapter 1   First things first 3

Chapter 2   Those dirty little secrets 11

Chapter 3   A big dilemma 17

Part II—Let's get real about meat, dairy and fish.

Chapter 4   Accelerated aging anyone?. 29

Chapter 5   How much and how often? 37

Chapter 6   Are you a baby cow? 47

Chapter 7   My, what small teeth you have. 57

Part III—Let's get real about starches, sweets and fats.

Chapter 8   Gluten, gluten and more gluten. 65

Chapter 9   Danger: Corn 75

Chapter 10 The great white witches, sugar and sweeteners.. . . 81

Chapter 11 What's in your fat? 89

Part IV—Let's get real about fruit, veggies, and water.

Chapter 12 Eat your fruits and veggies. 99

Chapter 13 Acid is for batteries 109

Chapter 14 Red, green and raw.. 117

Chapter 15 Clean water, please. 125

Part V—Let's get real about planning.

Chapter 16 Simple and not confused. 135

Final Words 145

The Rules from Let's Get Real about Eating 147

Sample Meal Plan 151

Bibliography and Resources 161

Endnotes 175

About the Author 191

Index 193

FOREWORD

"Look at what you put in your body." As I began my pediatric practice in 2006, this message resonated strongly within me. Since then, I have become more aware about the weaknesses in traditional pediatric training regarding nutrition. *Let's Get Real about Eating* will give you the knowledge about nutrition that 70-80% of pediatricians are lacking. The average physician did not learn during medical school or residency training what you will learn in this book. Knowledge and training in these areas of health and vitality are sought out by the practitioner independently and usually after their initial training.

Children are being diagnosed with disease processes at higher rates than ever before, and our next generation is taking as many or more medications than their parents. I am seeing parents who are scared to give their child medications prescribed by some of my colleagues. Medications, such as Methotrexate, Humera, Proton Pump Inhibitors, daily inhaled steroids, psychotropic medications and many, many more, are being infiltrated into our youngest patients. That is scary! Add the confusion experienced when you see TV shows featuring experts promoting foods and/or supplements to the inability of your doctors to discuss these valid alternatives with any real clarity and you have an abundance of unspoken fear, anger, and distrust. I ask myself as a physician, if I take this medication away or discontinue it, will the symptoms return? If the answer is yes, I have NOT done my job. To do my job well, I must also look at what my patients are putting into their bodies and educate them on the links between nutrition and disease that many doctors do not consider.

Let's Get Real about Eating helps you understand the underlying cause to many diseases. Understanding this gives you the knowledge and, hopefully, the motivation to view your family's healthcare needs differently. More than ever, disease is the result of poor nutrition. Poor nutrition has become habitual without understanding the imminent potential for disease. Don't let your worries, fear or even anger rest until you are sure you are doing everything you can to protect yourself and your children and ensure every measure is taken, so you and your children can live quality and independent lives. Reading this book is a great first step to get our children's health back—not to mention your own!

Sincere thanks to Laura Kopec for writing *Let's Get Real about Eating*. Even men, who are more a get-to-the point gender, will enjoy the simple rules and the bullet points in the "What Can You Do Right Now" segments. What you do NOW, matters! I don't want to sound like the pessimist, but if we do not change our nutrition, we will have to accept the healthcare costs that continue to rise, increasing treatments that have higher risk to the patient, and healthcare that does not address the root issues of most disease. This book will give you the confidence in the grocery store and give you the confidence when talking with your practitioner. You as the consumer must understand the financial relationships between the food industry and the government. This book makes it real and feasible to eat right while getting to the root of honest issues that many nutritionists will not address. Why? I wish I knew; but if we want anything to change in our health, we have to pay more attention to diet and lifestyle.

Thank you to Laura for keeping it simple, clear, and honest. This is not about being alternative or holistic or organic. It's about being "right" and speaking up about truth regarding our food. One of the best ways to speak up is by choosing the right, real foods.

I hope you, the reader, are one that recognizes the tides are changing in healthcare that this book will help steer the course for you, so that you can, "Look at what you put in your body."

Randy Naidoo, M.D.

ACKNOWLEDGEMENTS

I first would like to thank the health care professionals that have trusted me with their patients and allowing me the privilege of serving others and growing myself.

Thank you to Dr. Randy Naidoo, Dr. Homero Cavazos, Dr. Deborah Bain, and Dr. Sandy Gluckman for the time they have shared with me and what I have learned from each one.

I acknowledge and appreciate the many Moms I have worked with that are devoted to their own nutritional education in the pursuit of health for their children. They have greatly inspired me to reach more people with nutrition.

I am truly grateful to my editor, Anita Battista, for her input not only as an editor, but as a friend. Her candid feedback, as well as strong professionalism, is greatly appreciated.

Many supporters have read early chapters, notably Melissa Irvin,

Hillary Jarrard, Jennifer Goodman, Melanie Butts, Amy Hagg and Mariana Via. I am grateful to them for their support during this process.

A special thank you goes to Liza Orchard, Jerry Kopec, Marc Cook, and Pat Loewy for their loyalty and support.

Thank you to Dr. John DeMartini for his inspirational teachings. Thank you to Hawthorn University and a special thank you to Dr. Elizabeth Pavka.

I would like to thank Karimen Montero for all her help in this process, and her dedication to all that is Kopec Naturals.

Thank you to my dear friends Beverly Wells, Kari Berry, Tamara Crawford, and Alex Hyman for their support of my many journeys.

I would like to thank my children, Sierra, Luke and Eden for inspiring me to take the best care I can of their bodies, their minds and their hearts.

A Note to the Reader

The information in this book is provided to educate the reader on the health benefits of nutritional pursuits. However any decision involving the treatment of an illness should be made only after consulting a physician or health care practitioner of your choice. Neither this nor any book can guarantee complete absence of disease nor substitute professional medical care or treatment. The information contained in this book is not intended to serve as a replacement for professional medical advice. Any use of the information in this book is at the reader's discretion. The author and the publisher specifically disclaim any and all liability arising directly or indirectly from the use or application of any information contained in this book. A health care professional should be consulted regarding your specific situation. The client names have been eliminated in specific stories to protect their privacy.

INTRODUCTION

Everyday people of all ages and sizes come through my office, and I educate and coach them to make dietary changes that will improve their health. I have the good fortune to see many of these people make profound improvements in their health by changing what and how they eat. Typically one or more of the health issues listed at their first consultation include:

>> Digestive Complaints

>> Low Energy

>> Depression

>> Inflammation

>> Food Allergies and Sensitivities

>> Behavioral Disorders

>> Skin Conditions

Many people come to me when they have tried a variety of other paths and find no relief. Many individuals who incorporate what they have learned from me later report many symptoms are completely gone and their overall health is greatly improved. These changes occur because they make a decision to take charge of their health through nutrition. A young girl who suffered severe eczema came with her parents to see me. I educated Mom with dietary changes for her daughter, and with the dedication of Mom to make these changes, her daughter is completely free of eczema. The entire family is now dedicated to their overall health through good nutrition. I visited with the mom of a young boy who was diagnosed with autism. His parents came to me because he suffered from multiple food sensitivities. After providing his mother with a nutritional plan and nutritional guidance his mom noticed positive changes in his behavior, his speech and his social skills. A young woman came to me because she developed a facial rash while traveling overseas. After following a nutritional plan I created for her, not only did her rash go away, but a number of other issues she thought she would have for the rest of her life also went away. With changes like this possible for us all, I feel compelled to stand on the mountaintop and shout out the power of food. Every day I ask myself, how can I reach more people? How can I let everyone know the power of food? It seems almost too good to be true, that you can overcome some of your health issues by making dietary changes. It is true, and it *can* be done—especially when we understand the fundamentals of eating healthy.

I wrote this book to help more people understand just what we are missing when we discount the connection between what we eat and how we feel. I want you to know what has happened in this country to our food and how these changes in our food affect our health. Then, I want to simplify the issues and identify ways you can apply this knowledge in your own life. There is a lot of conflicting information out there about what to eat, what not to eat, when to eat, and how much to eat. This, in turn, makes the whole issue of nutrition and eating seem very confusing and too hard to tackle. There is a real need for a set of guidelines that provide some answers—simple and straightforward answers based on common sense, nature's laws and current research. I strive to give that set of guidelines to you in this book. Each chapter is packed with information that is summarized into a rule, and that rule is given a set of action steps to consider integrating into your daily life.

You can do the first few action steps listed in one or more chapters, or you can go all the way and do each and every step. It is up to you. Most people shy away from making changes to their diets because they believe it is either too hard, too expensive, or it is inconvenient to their lifestyle. What if I told you it is not necessary to give up the pleasure of eating in order to achieve optimal health? What if I told you that you could experience some results even if you want to do only some of what I suggest? Many people take baby steps, and still experience significant, positive changes in their health. I always say doing something is better than doing nothing, but also know that doing the most you can for your health, can bring about a quality of living you have never known.

Consider this. My grandmother said everything in moderation, and she was, for the most part, correct. The excessiveness in this country has become the root of most of our problems, including our health. As a result, we have lost the ability to know and understand the basic rules of nature that existed before we could buy anything any time of the day or night. Obesity, diabetes, cancer, heart disease, gastrointestinal disorders, ADD, ADHD, celiac disease, food allergies and sensitivities, autoimmune, inflammation are all on the rise. We have to make some changes in the way we eat and the way we live, or we will find the list of chronic and degenerative diseases growing beyond what our health care is able to manage. Each year in the United States alone, an estimated 565,000 people have their first heart attack, 1.3 million adults are diagnosed with diabetes, and 1.4 million develop cancer.[1] Those numbers should scare many of us, but they do not. We continue to eat and eat ourselves into a state of crisis. In 1960, the World Health Organization found most cancer to be preventable with better nutrition,[2] and we still have yet to make cancer a disease of the past. Dr. Michael McGinnis, a well-known public servant and

Senior Scholar at the Institute of Medicine, has stated that diet is the number two killer of Americans;[3] but not only do we refuse to change, most parents are letting their children fall into worse eating habits than they themselves have. As a result, this upcoming generation of children may have a shorter life span over their parents.[4] If we will not do this for ourselves, will we do this for our children?

The time to do something is now. Even if you are not ready for a complete change of lifestyle, do something. Some change is better than no change, especially given how far we have strayed. Right now, I challenge you to get real about the way you eat and your children eat, and do something. Take action. Take charge of your health by eating for your health; and when you eat better, you will feel better.

Baby steps are a necessary part of dietary changes; otherwise, changes may not be permanent. Let this book be a starting place, both in understanding and in action, to help us make sense of it all. If we can begin those crucial steps without feeling overwhelmed, then we can begin to feel good again, because feeling good really is only a forkful away.

PART I

Let's get real about additives, pesticides, and GMO's.

"Vitality and beauty are gifts of Nature for
those who live according to its laws."
—Leonardo Da Vinci

CHAPTER ONE

First things first

WHEN I SPEAK in front of large groups of people and talk about the dangers of the current American diet there is always the question, "What should I change first?" It is a fair question. There is so much information regarding nutrition and such differing opinions about what we should eat and what we should give up, that it really is hard to know what your first step should be. In the face of such differing opinions and confusing do's and don'ts the first step should be manageable. This first step is an easy concept, not always easy to put into practice, but profoundly positive to your health. Eat real food. Real food is food that grows in nature, on trees, in the ground, or was once a living breathing animal. Real food does not contain chemical or artificial ingredients.

Why should we eat real food? A great analogy is a car. A car runs on gasoline. An automobile would not run well if you put rocks in the gas tank. Our bodies are similar machines that run on a certain kind of fuel. If we put chemical ingredients or artificial ingredients in our body it is as if we have put rocks in our gas tank. Ultimately the magnificent machine known as the human body will suffer consequences of putting rocks in our gas tank. Put another way, the human body is most comfortable digesting food that it recognizes to be similar to its own makeup. Ingredients unrecognizable such as artificial colors and flavors can cause the immune system to respond as if the body is being invaded.[5] The unrecognizable ingredients that engage the immune system are essentially toxic to the human body. The human body then determines how to deal with these invaders/ toxins and so begins illness and disease. Determining what is real and what is toxic to our health is actually becoming more and more confusing, so in this next section I will share with you some of the hard facts about what we are really putting in our mouths. It is not a pretty picture.

Many of us make decisions in the grocery store based on what we can afford and what tastes good, or might be interesting to our family. Very few of us are thinking about whether or not what we are eating is actually good for us. Over seventeen thousand new "food" products hit the grocery stores every year and this is very confusing for the average consumer.[6] How are we expected to stay on top of all the new food items hitting our shelves? The truth is you don't have to stay on top of all the so-called advancements in food practices, but you do have to take ownership of the real reason your body needs to eat (energy and nutrients), and then you need to know how to read a label. Many packaged foods are meant to tempt to our taste buds and appeal to us on many different levels, keeping us from stepping back and taking a real look at the product's nutritional content. But since four out of ten deaths in this country are associated with poor eating habits,[7] it is imperative we learn how to move through a grocery store and how to read our labels.

If you are looking at your food labels, chances are you are paying attention to calories, or maybe grams of sugar or maybe sodium. If so, you are missing a huge piece to the puzzle: the list of ingredients.

This is the most telling section of your label. The list may begin with ingredients such as enriched wheat flour and then list other ingredients such as high fructose corn syrup. Your list may be as long as five or twenty-five different ingredients. Currently over twelve thousand different ingredients are used in the manufacturing of food,[8] and it is safe to say nature did not give us all twelve thousand. The FDA is involved in approving what ingredients get to go into your food. They have approved real preservatives such as ascorbic acid (a naturally occurring compound otherwise known as vitamin C) and cochineal (a red dye derived from the cochineal insect), but the FDA also approves artificial ingredients like Erythrosine, otherwise known as red dye #3, which has been linked to thyroid tumors in rats.[9] Tocopherol, a seemingly complicated word is actually Vitamin E, but sodium benzoate, which is often found in salad dressings, carbonated drinks and fruit juices, is also considered rocket fuel. When sodium benzoate combines with vitamin C, it is a carcinogen, so the FDA allows only a small amount to be used in food. A small amount may be considered safe by the FDA, but should you consider it safe enough for your health? You could say when we eat these foods we are playing with fire, and you would not be too far off.

Let's take a look at one particular type of artificial ingredient: food dyes and let's consider what they might be doing to our health, especially the health of our children. To begin with, more and more research links negative behaviors, such as attention disorders, hyperactivity and the inability to sit still with ingesting food dyes.[10] Dr. Feingold, a noted pediatrician practicing between the late 1920's until the late 70's discovered there was a real problem for many children who consumed food dyes establishing a link between the new chemicals in food and certain behaviors. His findings were considered radical at the time, but have won over many since, including many of his own critics. By the 1980's many researchers gave his initial findings serious consideration. Then in 2007, a formal study was conducted which involved the Food Advisory Committee and the FDA. The FDA stated there was no reason to advise the consumer of the potential dangers of food dyes until a more in depth (expensive) study is conducted.[11] Should we wait until the tests have been completed? Should we trust our government to put our health first? Other countries are not waiting.

The British Foods Standard Agency advised their consumers, especially parents to eliminate food colorings from the diets of children.[12] As of 2010, the European Union requires a warning label on all foods containing artificial colors of the potential adverse effect on children's activity and attention.[13] Companies such as Kellogg®, McDonald's®, Kraft®, and Mars® all have removed food dyes from the products they ship to Great Britain and Europe, but continue to give the food dyes to consumers in the United States.[14] We really should not wait for further testing. We should not wait for manufacturers to do the right thing. We have to become more aware and read labels. We can use our common sense to help us navigate through the grocery store, read labels with true understanding, and know without a shadow of a doubt what food is nourishing to our body, and which ingredients are suspect.

The first step is to eat foods that will rot, go bad, grow mold or attract bugs. This may turn you off since many of us want our food to last a long time, but it is essential. I had a client come to me for nutritional counseling, and she learned a great deal about eating real food and was so excited to add more fresh fruits and vegetables into her diet. But after one month of fresh produce in the house, she could not stand the fruit flies in her kitchen, and she was very tempted to go back to snacks in a box. My advice to her was to make sure all produce was stored in the refrigerator when the weather was warmer and to keep counters clean of food particles. The real food she was feeding her family had brought about such amazing changes in their overall health that it wasn't worth quitting over something that could be solved fairly simply. Many of us like the convenience of packaged food because it can sit out on the counter, and we don't have to make a weekly trip to the grocery store. The result being that many of us are paying such severe health consequences in exchange for less frequent trips to the grocery store and don't even realize it. There are definite adjustments when we start to eat more real food, but let's take a hard look at what food with extended shelf life might be doing to our bodies.

Our digestive systems are designed to break down decomposable foods. Most processed foods are designed to keep from breaking down, so that they can sit on the shelf for an extended period of time. The human body needs food that decomposes quickly, so it can extract nutrients from this food as it breaks down which in turn fuels and nourishes our bodies. Food that is designed to sit on the shelf in the grocery store and our pantries for an extended period of time does not decompose readily. If you really think about it, what kind of chance does your stomach have with a food designed to sit on the shelf for an extended period of time versus food that is prone to decompose?

The stomach produces acid for protein breakdown and to help destroy unwanted bacteria and prepare food for the small intestine to absorb. When food is either too difficult to break down, or will not readily decompose the stomach may be confused and may make too much or too little stomach acid. Too little or too much stomach acid may result in heartburn. For many people, heartburn is not too much acid, but the result of too little stomach acid which results in poor protein breakdown and further malabsorption in the small intestines. Heartburn may then lead to further health issues such as obesity, irritable bowel syndrome, and dyspepsia.[15] Many individuals address heartburn with an antacid. Stomach acid is needed for nutrient break down, but when we suppress the discomfort of heartburn with antacid, we may consequently suppress one of our body's necessary functions. Your heartburn may be a serious warning from your body that it is time to change your diet.

Changing the diet begins with being able to understand real food and how to read a label. The first group of real food has *no* ingredient label. The food *is* the ingredient. For example, a banana has no ingredient list it is just itself. It is real food. Anything that does not need an ingredient label, carrots, eggs, broccoli, apples, is real food. For most of us, understanding whole foods such as bananas and carrots is fairly simple, but it is when we get into packaged food that the trouble begins. You need to know two things. One, you need to know how to pronounce the ingredient. Don't eat it if you cannot pronounce it. But we cannot stop there, because manufacturers are renaming some of our problem ingredients to simpler names that are easy to pronounce. So, more importantly than pronouncing it alone—if you do not know how the ingredient *came to be*, how it was grown, or made, then don't eat it. An example of this is soy protein isolate. Easy to pronounce, so it must be okay? Do you know how to make soy protein isolate? Do you know how it came to be? Can you make it in your kitchen? Are you willing to take a chance that it could be derived from a natural source, or is it better to be as safe as you possibly can be? Assume these ingredients are guilty first, until you know otherwise. After all it is your health that matters.

A young woman came to my office for nutritional counseling for her teenage son. He had been in the hospital with headaches and stomach issues and had to drop out of the remainder of the school semester. None of the many specialists he saw considered that what he was eating and drinking on a regular basis may have been a factor in his poor health. After finding out he was drinking a particular sports drink in large quantities and ate a diet of processed foods, almost never eating a fresh fruit or vegetable it was time to make a change. Within a month of eating real foods as part of a customized nutritional plan, his health showed tremendous improvement. You don't have to be in the hospital to decide to make a change. You don't have to be without hope from the medical establishment to make a change. You can just decide it is time to take charge of your eating.

Now that you have some good information, you need a plan and some real strategies that will help you put this information into practice and make some good choices that profoundly affect your health. Below is your first rule to help guide you. The rule is followed by a list of action strategies to help you put the rule into practice. You can do one step, or you can do all the steps. You may do a few steps for a while and once you feel comfortable advance to doing more. You decide.

RULE # 1: EAT REAL FOOD.

What you can do right now:

1. Take ownership. The only way to stay committed to eating better quality food is to make a commitment to your health and to the real reasons your body eats. Fuel and nutrients.

2. Trust no one. You should not trust your government, the media, or a third party organization to make the best decisions for your packaged foods. You can use your own common sense to help guide you through the grocery stores.

3. Read what is in your pantry. Many of us do not even realize what we have been eating, so the first step is to become aware of what is on your label. Can you pronounce it? Can you understand it? Do you know how the ingredient was made? Do you really want to put something into your very own body when you do not know where it came from?

4. Be smart. Fill your grocery cart with lots of *single* ingredient foods like carrots, bananas, eggs, apples, and almonds. At least 2/3 of your grocery cart should be single ingredient foods.

5. Add smart. Add at least one single ingredient food at every meal. Example, add a banana or blueberries to your breakfast cereal. If you have yogurt, add fruit. If you have eggs, add tomato or onion.

6. Think smart. Shop the old fashioned way. Imagine yourself at a farmer's market while in the grocery store, and purchase the majority of your groceries *as if* from the farm. The places around the world with the best health have no access to processed food, eating a plethora of whole foods. We do not have to live on the farm to be healthy, but we should grocery shop as if we do.

7. Be language savvy. When shopping, remember it is not just about the pronunciation of an ingredient. It is also about understanding how the ingredient came to be.

8. Choose one. Begin with one artificial ingredient and phase out of the buying of this ingredient. Start with artificial colors. Eliminate the food dyes.

9. Take a stand. Refuse to buy products from companies such as Kellogg®, McDonald's®, Kraft®, and Mars® that removed food dyes out of the food they ship overseas, but not in the United States.

10. Shop weekly. Eating real food means you may have to increase the frequency with which you go to the grocery store. Many places around the world have to go to an open market every day for their food, but we do not have this luxury. Many of us in this country are too busy to go to market everyday. If you think about it a weekly trip is not such a bad thing.

11. Health matters. Remember what you eat impacts your health, and the quality of your life is greatly improved when you feel better.

12. Don't give up. When making the transition to eating better it is easy to feel frustrated and want to give up, especially if you are a Mom and cannot get your family on board with eating better. When feeling discouraged, remind yourself that you care about your health and the health of your children. These are great reasons to stay dedicated.

CHAPTER TWO

Those dirty little secrets

W HEN I ASK a brand new client what their biggest objection is to making nutritional changes the answer often is nutrition is too confusing, and the second biggest obstacle is the belief that eating healthy is too expensive. Many people believe that eating healthy means eating everything organic. And organic is more money. The idea of spending more on groceries is such a threatening idea to so many that they give up before they even start because they cannot buy organic. You can still make profound changes in your health by following Chapter One and eating real food whether it is organic or not. Real food will always take precedent because it is nature given. Eating real food is your first step, but in your quest for optimal health, you should know all the facts about food, and that includes whether or not you should buy organic. In this chapter, I want to raise your awareness of organic versus conventional food, of the true nature of pesticides, what kind of pesticides you are exposed to, and how you can have good strategies for grocery shopping that will fit your health and budget.

Pesticide is the term given to a substance used to control, destroy, repel or even attract a pest. They were introduced to farming in the 1940's and continue to be used as the main agriculture practice for controlling and destroying pests. Pesticides were openly used to help farmers increase their yield by controlling the pest population. Then about twenty years later, suspicion as to their safety arose. Some pesticides were found to be "harmful," but only those found to be "very harmful" were subsequently banned from the United States. Pesticides have been linked to numerous conditions involving many of the body's systems. Some of these conditions include infertility, abnormal sperm, even birth defects. Pesticides have been linked to thyroid issues and adrenal fatigue. In some cases, pesticides have been linked to cancer.[16]

In the United States, we use approximately one billion pounds of pesticides every year. Each individual in this country consumes approximately three pounds of the billion.[17] Many of these pesticides are indirectly ingested through the flesh of a fruit or vegetable, or in the grains and other foods we consume. The Environmental Protection Agency (EPA) lists 107 different ingredients in pesticides as carcinogens. The EPA lists another entire class of pesticides as nerve toxins, and then another entire category of pesticides as poisons. Seventy of these 107 are used on food crops.[18] It doesn't even make sense that we would be exposed to such high level toxins, but they are in fact in our food supply. Pesticides continue to be used in spite of their health consequences. Pesticides are linked to lung cancer, pancreatic, colon and rectal cancers, all lymph cancers, leukemia, non-Hodgkin lymphoma, breast, bladder, and prostate cancer, brain, melanoma and childhood cancers and yet we continue to use pesticides by the tons.[19]

There are many troubling facts surrounding the use of pesticides, but the most disturbing fact is our current consumption of illegal and banned pesticides. How does this happen? It goes like this. The United

States ships 110,000 tons of pesticides to other countries. Many of these pesticides that we ship abroad are the very same ones that are banned in this country. Once the banned pesticide is exported to other countries they use these illegal pesticides on their produce, and then import this produce back into the United States for our consumption. In fact, half of the imported produce tested in this country, tests positive for illegal pesticides.[20] This means we have no real regulations against the ingestion of illegal pesticides. We can only say we ban them in this country, we cannot say we are not consuming them. Other concerning pesticides have restrictions on how much a farmer can use, but some states such as California have tested in excess of the safe amount of restricted pesticides. In 1995, an EPA restricted use pesticide known as methyl bromide was reported in excess of 17 million pounds used in California on fruits such as grapes and strawberries. Metam sodium, an EPA labeled carcinogen, was reported by the California Department of Agriculture to have been used in excess of 15 million pounds.[21] While rampant consumption of pesticides exist there continues to be damages often unspoken by the average person, that of the environment.

Consequences to the environment such as groundwater contamination, crop loss, bird, fish and other animal deaths are linked to pesticide exposure along with damage to the population of bees. These environmental damages cost taxpayers billions and billions of dollars annually.[22] There is also a growing fear that we have bred super insects that are pesticide resistant and therefore highly damaging to crops. In a recent conversation with an agriculture professor, I learned that we cannot completely eliminate the use of pesticides globally otherwise the modern insect, which is more powerful than previous generations of insects, would wipe out many of our crops leaving our food supply in jeopardy. We cannot escape simple facts such as the permanent damage of our pesticide use, and we have to suffer the consequences. But as consumers we can still navigate successfully and make the best choices we can for our families and ourselves.

Thanks to groups such as The Environmental Working Group (EWG), a non-profit organization dedicated to consumers, you and

I can be educated on how to navigate through the grocery store more affectively when it comes to pesticides. EWG reviews produce annually and puts out a report ranking the produce with the highest amount of pesticide residue along with those testing the cleanest. This list can help consumers plan and prioritize which foods are the most contaminated with pesticides. This way we can save some money if we cannot buy exclusively organic by avoiding the most contaminated or the most dangerous of foods. Avoiding highly contaminated fruits and vegetable along with avoiding imported produce are steps we the consumer can take to make a difference in our lives and the world we live in.

Gandhi said, "Be the change you want in the world." We need to take a stand as consumers in the grocery store. Otherwise, we cannot expect our agriculture practices to ever change. Each time we buy organic, we send a message to farmers that we want organic produce, and we are willing to pay the difference. Think about this. You can pay for produce grown safely upfront, bearing the cost of organic produce, while doing something to help influence the status quo and experiencing improved health that will likely lower the overall cost of your own and your family's health care. Or your taxes can continue to pay for the environmental damages and rising healthcare issues with your personal blessing, and you can pay physically and emotionally in health consequences for you or your family members, not to mention the money you will spend on the health issues you and your children acquire from pesticide consumption. You choose.

Rule #2: Avoid buying and eating food with high levels of pesticide residue.

What you can do right now:

1. Know the code. Organic produce is labeled with a small sticker beginning with the number 9. Conventional, non-organic produce that may contain pesticide residue begins with the

number 4. Make sure your produce is labeled correctly, no matter what the store advertises.

2. Shop the farmer's market. When you make a trip to the farmer's market, you get to look a real person in the eye and ask them what they are using on their produce. Some farmer's will tell you they use organic measures to prevent insects which may be the same measure certified organics use. Some will tell you they are using standard or conventional measures to help control the insect population, and then it is up to you. You can also see if there is the tell-tale sticker betraying the produce was actually purchased and brought to the market under the guise of local and fresh, which unfortunately has happened to me on a few occasions. Once I had a lengthy conversation where a woman behind the table talked about her beautiful plum orchard, and then upon closer inspection I saw the grocery store sticker upon which she had to admit she had purchased the plums.

3. Be in the know. Check out the Environmental Working Group's website www.ewg.org and view their current report on which fruit and vegetables have the highest trace of pesticides.

4. Avoid imported produce. Whether you buy organic or not, you need to avoid conventional produce from other countries. Remember—we sell illegal pesticides. Other countries use it on their crops. They import back to the United States. You do the math.

5. Protect your home. While the majority of pesticide exposure comes from food, other sources include what we use in our backyard and insect repellants. Websites such as www. organicgardening.com gives you great tips on how to care for your backyard organically.

6. Wash your produce. Wash fruits and vegetables under warm water and a scrub brush. If you want to get fancy, you can make a solution using 8-10 oz. of water and a few drops of

oregano essential oil or a few drops of liquid grapefruit seed extract in a spray bottle. Spray your produce, scrub and rinse clean. Even though we cannot wash away the pesticides that have permeated the flesh of our fruits and vegetables, we should still wash any residue on the outside along with any unwanted organisms or bacteria.

7. Plant a garden. If buying organic is too much of an expense, try planting a few vegetables in your own garden. It doesn't have to be big, just a few tomatoes and peppers will help you reduce your cost of organic produce and help you appreciate how vegetables are grown. If you cannot grow a garden on your property, you could talk to your local church and see if they have the same restrictions. If not, suggest a church-sponsored community garden where volunteers can participate in the growing, and the church can sell or donate baskets to their members. Or try container gardening. Tomatoes, zucchini, strawberries and herbs make great container plants. Herbs will even grow indoors with success.

CHAPTER THREE

A big dilemma

I HAVE BEEN RESEARCHING nutrition since 1995, and never has a topic been so challenging as genetically modified food. So many of the nutritional books I own fail to even examine the topic. After all, it is a highly charged topic that easily leads to overwhelming issues like global hunger, poor research, consumer ignorance and governmental apathy. It is easy to get tied up in one aspect of the issues and lose sight of the biggest issue—no one knows enough to know for sure if genetically modified food is safe for consumption, much less as a solution to global hunger issues.

According to Jeffrey Smith (a leading activist against genetically modified food) many activists, scientists, environmentalists and farmers believe the appropriate studies to determine the true safety of genetically modified food have not even been done.[23] Instead, the large companies manufacturing the genetically modified organisms (GMO) used in many foods want us to believe that the initial studies proved no further testing is really necessary and that genetically modified food is the answer to global starvation and global warming.

The very idea that eventually every person on the planet could be eating food containing genetically modified organisms should be reason enough to do all the research and studies necessary to remove any doubt this is safe to eat. I consider myself not only a holistic nutritionist but also an environmentalist, and when presented with the choice between my own health and whether or not children around the world would be fed, my head spins. Michael Pollan, noted food expert and author of books such as *Food Rules,* put this so well in his *NY Times* article against genetically modified rice when he said it appears, "…if we don't get over our queasiness about eating genetically modified food, kids in the third world will [suffer]."[24] He too believed initially that he had to accept genetically modified foods or children in underdeveloped countries would starve. Once he understood that genetically modified food was not the answer to starvation, he no longer had the conflict between what he believed to be nutritionally sound and his compassion for others. This chapter examines the multiple controversies surrounding genetically modified food, the potential health risks associated with eating genetically modified food, and whether or not we should trust the food we eat.

Genetically modified food is food that contains one or more genetically modified organisms (GMO). This means that the food crop in its original form, such as corn, now contains DNA different from the original DNA that nature provided. Often the crop is given supporting genes along with the new genes to help the plant DNA not reject the newly added DNA. Then when the genetically modified crop reproduces, the added genes are automatically in the new seeds which will grow according to their altered genetic makeup. Greenpeace, a widely recognized nonprofit organization promoting the protection of the environment, calls this contamination of our food crops "genetic manipulation" that becomes "genetic pollution."[25]

Once the DNA of the crop has been altered, the crop can be patented and sold at a profit. This kind of profit-making scenario can only be recognized as a huge motivator behind the massive food production containing genetically modified organisms. Without the ability to patent and profit, it is quite possible there would be more truth and less controversy about GMO's. Instead, genetically modified food is here, and it accounts for a significant part of what we are eating on a daily basis. Given the amount of genetically modified food already in production, what does the average person need to know?

Large corporations manufacturing genetically modified food want you to believe that GMO, prepares to feed a growing global population, benefits starving populations now, and minimizes the effects of global weather changes. It is true that there is an impending crisis of need due to these issues. The global population of 6.9 billion in 2012 is expected to reach 9 billion by 2050; and in order to sustain this growth, food production has to increase by 50%.[26] In addition, a significant percentage of the current global population is starving. Over 925 million people worldwide are hungry. The large majority, approximately 578 million, are hungry in Asia and the Pacific. Another 276 million people are hungry in Africa.[27] To further complicate the issue of world hunger, global weather patterns are changing. According to the Environmental Protection Agency (EPA), temperature changes and increased rainfall brought on temperature changes could have a positive effect on how fast crops will grow but a negative affect on crop yields. The 2008 flood in the Mississippi region reported a loss of 8 billion dollars by farmers, and across the states livestock owners report losses of approximately 5,000 animals from heat waves.[28] A Stanford study proposes that there would have been an increase in both wheat and corn production since 1980 had it not been for climate changes. [29]

Take world hunger; despite the fact that large companies promoting GMOs believe GMOs are the answer to global hunger, research on world hunger claims that an increase in crop production has *never* been the answer to feeding the hungry.[30] In 2005, 934 million people did not have access to developing land. Studies conducted by the Global Land Tool Network and UN–Habitat demonstrate that access to land improves food security, stimulates economic growth and increases the number of people that go without struggle in these areas.[31] Those without access to land as well as many others lack the means and education necessary to provide for themselves and their families by other means. Poverty and lack of education, not lack of food, appear to be the main reason people go hungry. If people were given access to developing land and we taught them gardening, animal husbandry or other ways to be more self-sustainable in areas of little land, we would address the main reasons why people go hungry. OxFam, an international confederation of seventeen organizations that stand for global change against hunger, takes no position on the health of GMO's, but does firmly believe GMO's are not the solution to hunger and poverty.[32]

The next issue is a growing population. The debate on whether or not genetically modified crops feeds a growing population has been disputed by a variety of experts that say there is no scientific research, only marketing analysis, that supports increased crop yields. In fact, many scientific experts actually argue lower yield by genetically modified crops.[33] An even bigger issue than lower yield is farmers' complaints of an inability to grow healthy crops after their fields were "infected" with genetically modified crops.[34]

Additional research in favor of genetically modified food claims crops are being designed to be drought resistant. Some of these crops have been reported to help countries like Africa, which has suffered its worst droughts in recent years.[35] But the research being conducted at Stanford claims that heavy and unpredictable rainfall is a more significant problem in some areas over the lack of rainfall.[36] The question regarding whether or not GMO is the answer to weather changes remains to be seen, but if farmers are complaining about crop yields and the ability to grow at all once genetically modified crops have been planted and weather changes are affecting yields, it does not appear genetically modified crops will prove to be the total solution to weather changes. Genetically modified crops are not a global solution and should be questioned as a healthy solution to any of the related issues.

What does the American consumer need to know about the health and safety of GMOs? First you need to know that our food is not adequately labeled. You don't know what you are eating. There is sheer disregard for informing us about which foods are genetically modified foods. Unless you are eating food that you grow yourself from seeds that have not been genetically altered or you live in a self-sustaining community with no infrastructure, then chances are very great you are eating genetically modified food. If we are going to eat it, shouldn't we know it? Currently there is no regulation requiring a manufacturer to label their food product as containing genetically modified organisms.[37] Without proper labeling how are we to know what we are eating?

According to Greenpeace, profits are behind the public being kept in the dark about which food products contain genetically modified organisms.[38] Many states are petitioning to have labeling laws placed on the ballot so the general public can vote to have food labeled as containing genetically modified organisms. While these efforts are a great step in the right direction, they will take time before the consumer sees this kind of labeling, if the petitions are successful and the vote is in favor. In the meantime, a non-profit organization called "Non-GMO Project" is an independent verification program helping manufacturers label their food to be free of genetically modified organisms.[39] This is an important first step to helping the consumer know what is in their food. Right now, the most common genetically modified crops are corn, potatoes, canola, soybeans, papayas, and squash.[40] As consumers, we should know whether or not these crops line our produce shelves or become part of packaged foods. If there is no problem with genetically modified food, then accurate labeling should not hurt anyone.

The next biggest problem with genetically modified food is the potential for tremendous health risks. In a monumental gathering of data, *Genetic Roulette,* Jeffrey Smith examines health risks associated with genetically modified food such as infertility, cancer, increase in food allergies, DNA mutations, altered levels of nutrients, damage to kidneys and livers, increase risk of disease, potential for unhealthy embryo development and even death.[41] Most intriguingly, the data revealed that cows, pigs, deer, mice and other animals, when given the choice between genetically modified food and non-genetically modified food, chose the non-genetically modified food.[42] Animals by instinct are avoiding these kinds of food, but too often we are eating these foods without even a choice. The health problems associated with the consumption of genetically modified food is becoming more and more apparent, so at the very least we should have a choice. Instead, large companies with profits at stake keep us in the dark.

Companies behind the pro-GMO research are companies such as Mosanto, responsible for 88% of the genetically modified crops planted today.[43] The money invested by Mosanto, and the profits to be made by this company makes their studies biased. They have significant conflict of interest, and in independents studies, their research has been proven to be flawed.[44] Mosanto has often been accused of contradicting itself, and even though follow up studies from around the world have been requested, none have been conducted.[45] Research conducted by companies with profit interests combined with contradictions should not be considered credible research. Less than a dozen animal safety studies and one human study account for all the scientific research of the genetically modified food we are eating every day.[46] One scientist in particular, Arpaid Pusztai of the Rowlett Research Institute, dared to conduct an independent study, speak publicly of his results and demand that more research be conducted. He was subsequently fired and his research was seized.[47] His team had conducted a study of genetically modified potatoes and their effect on the health of rats. Pusztai's experiments showed the rats to have immune system damage along with precancerous cells, and damage to their brains and their livers.[48] Even after being fired, Pusztai continues to speak out on the internet regarding his views of genetically modified food.

Not only are scientists who risk their jobs and reputations, like Pusztai, helping us understand the dangers of genetically modified food, but lawsuits that helped make FDA files public record also are big eye openers. One filed by the Alliance of Biointegrity resulted in more than 20 different files being made public. These files revealed concerns by FDA scientists themselves on the safety of food containing genetically modified organisms.[49] In the document entitled Revision of Toxicology Section of the *Statement of Policy: Foods Derived from Genetically Modified Plants* dated January 31, 1992, Dr. Samuel I. Shibko stated to Dr. James Maryansksi, FDA Biotechnology Coordinator, "FDA believes that...the possibility of unexpected, accidental changes in genetically engineered plants justifies a limited traditional toxicological study."[50] This means enough of a problem was discovered to demand further testing.

The very idea that these organisms pose potential or real dangers to us and yet are still a major part of food production with no further studies in the works is unbelievable and disheartening. At the very least, labeling should be mandatory. Whether you stand for technological advancement in food production or believe there are dire consequences for altering nature, the bottom line is there is not enough conclusive evidence to indicate without a shadow of a doubt genetically modified food is safe and harmless for human consumption. We need to keep ourselves educated. We need to demand better labeling. We need to know what is in our food. Let's keep ourselves and our children from being the experiment.

Rule #3: Know your food, especially the genetically modified stuff.

1. Know the list. As of August 2012, the food crops containing genetically engineered organisms are: alfalfa, corn, canola, soybeans, papayas, zucchini and crook neck squash. Potatoes and tomatoes are no longer genetically modified. There is a strain of rice genetically modified called golden rice, but this is primarily grown and sold in the Philippines and Taiwan. Sugar cane and salmon are next to be genetically modified. Currently, in order to avoid GMO versions of these foods, you must buy organic.

2. Buy organic. Make sure you buy these foods and food ingredients as organic to ensure they are not genetically modified: corn, sugar, soy, and canola. This includes foods like canola oil, corn syrup, soybean oil, soy lecithin, and even cane sugar can be GMO unless organic.

3. Be afraid. As long as the research shows the potential for a variety of health risks, we should be worried for our health, the health of the animals we eat and the health of our children.

4. Question the source. We live in a world of information overload. All too often we take information at face value. Private companies with profit interests in the outcome of research should not be allowed to conduct the research. As a consumer, you can refuse to accept research by profit motivated companies.

5. Check it out. The NON-GMO Project website (http://www.nongmoproject.org) has a lot of great information about what brands voluntarily participate in labeling their products to be non-GMO.

6. Support non-GMO. You can support businesses that are conscious about avoiding genetically modified organisms. You can also support local farmers that avoid using seeds containing genetically modified organisms. Take a trip to your local farmer's market and talk directly to your local farmers. Find out their position, and their practices.

7. Plant an heirloom garden. Heirloom seeds are labeled as such. Heirloom means the seed is the original seed without any kind of genetic modification or alteration. Seeds of Change® is a reputable company providing heirloom seeds to the consumer. When you grow a garden, you create a deeper appreciation of and connection to the food you eat, and it is healthy way to learn more about growing practices.

8. Donate a goat. Go online and buy a goat or a chicken for a starving family in Africa. When you help provide food and

an income source in the form of a goat or chicken you help a family become more self-sufficient and help reduce their poverty. Organizations such as World of Vision, Hands of Hope, Compassion International, and Heifer International help make this possible. Global Giving, Plan USA and Women for Women International also give opportunities to help strengthen and support impoverished countries. If we all took small steps to help provide alternative means of feeding our hungry, we would be helping hungry populations avoid GMO crops as a main source of food.

9. Sign a petition. If you live in a state with an active petition to get GMO labeling on the ballot, sign it. Better labeling laws may very well inspire a movement for better testing on genetically modified foods. The website "Just Label It!" (http://justlabelit.org/) is seeking signatures to petition the FDA for better labeling. Better labeling is important for us all.

PART II

Let's get real about meat, dairy and fish.

"A man too busy to take care of his health is like a
mechanic too busy to take care of his tools."
—Spanish Proverb

CHAPTER FOUR

Accelerated aging anyone?

$\mathcal{I}$N THIS COUNTRY we like our meat. It is almost always the center of our meals. Anytime I ask someone what they are having for dinner they reply, "Chicken" or "Meatloaf" or "Salmon." No one ever says, "Spinach and asparagus with salmon on the side." It is our focus and our nature to desire meat. Even our restaurants are centered on meat. Burger joints, wings, steak houses, ribs, and fast food. Animal protein is an essential source of protein, vitamin B12, amino acids and iron; yet while meat is a staple to most Americans, it is luxury in many places around the world. Most Americans are spoiled. We refuse to see meat as a luxury item and want to pay as little as possible for it. The demand for inexpensive meat often results in poor quality meat, which is now costing us our health. The truth is we need to improve the quality of our meat if we are going to keep it at the center of our meals. Unless we do so, we will continue to pay tremendous health consequences. This chapter will examine two of the main concerns about eating meat in this country, and why we need to change the quality of the meat we eat.

The average consumer in the United States consumes vast quantities of hormone contaminated meat, dairy and eggs. If diet-related illness and disease were not so prevalent in this country, we could turn a blind eye to the fact of growth hormones in food. We can no longer avoid this ugly truth. We spend billions of dollars on wrinkle creams and plastic surgery proving that holding onto our youth is important to us, but how many of us have been told that some basic food items such as meat and dairy could be aging us prematurely. Growth hormones essentially accelerate the growth of the animal in order to maximize profits, but accelerated growth is really accelerated aging. And when the animal is given growth hormones, it becomes part of the meat or the milk and then we consume the growth hormones.

Consuming growth hormones that accelerate the growth and aging of the animal means we are accelerating our own aging. (Hopefully I have just appealed to your vanity and you are sitting up and taking notice). We definitely don't want to grow old before our time. And I, for one, don't want our children to either. You agree? Eating food contaminated with growth hormones is potentially a real crisis for children. The consumption of growth hormones has been linked to early puberty[51] and on the surface it seems harmless enough. But early puberty is now associated with an increased risk for breast and prostate cancer. In fact, the rate of breast cancer is three times higher in girls who started puberty before the age of twelve.[52] It is time to take a stand for ourselves and our children and it begins with taking a look at some of these chemicals.

Progesterone, testosterone, zeranol, trebolone, melengestrol, oestrogen, oestradiol are some of the names of the hormones given to cattle. In December of 2000, The National Toxicology Program named oestrogen as a carcinogen and the Environmental Protection Agency (EPA) named oestrogen as unsafe.[53] The Scientific Committee of Veterinary Medicine reported these hormones to be linked to developmental, immunological, neurobiological, immunotoxic and carcinogenic effects.[54] These are some serious concerns. A 1980 confidential report submitted to the FDA shows excessive levels of hormones in meat.[55] It is maddening to think our entire population could be suffering from consuming high levels of growth hormones.

The United States stands very loosely on policies surrounding growth hormones in food, but the European Union thinks differently and stands firm on their policies. Using the Scientific Committee's report, the European Union placed a ban on synthetic hormones in meat and even asked that naturally occurring hormones be used only for therapeutic purposes.[56] Interestingly enough, when the European Union placed this ban on synthetic hormones in meat, this in turn restricted imported meats containing these hormones. The United States was a significant supplier of beef to Europe at the time, but the ban now placed the United States supply of meat in jeopardy. Europe refused to import beef from the United States into its countries. In retaliation, the United States created a tariff on European imports such as wine, cheese and olive oil. This tax costs Europeans approximately $116.8 million annually. To make sure the tax would be an ongoing penalty the United States established the contract to renew itself every six months.[57] The European government stays firm on their policies surrounding imported foods despite the cost to them and feels the sacrifice of millions of dollars has greater impact on the health of their citizens. It would be beneficial if the United States took time to rethink current policies on meat production beginning with the diet of the animal.

Many animals that will eventually wind up on our tables have a very poor diet. Many of these animals are overweight and sick. This is not surprising. Many animals that eat a grain-based diet have difficulty digesting and tend to carry extra weight due to growth hormones, diet and lack of mobility. Obesity in an animal means there is a greater amount of fat. A greater amount of fat means there is a greater capacity for the animals to store toxins since toxins are stored in the fatty tissue of living animals. This means we, the consumer, have a greater chance of ingesting the animals' toxins and increasing the toxic load on our own body.

A higher concentration of fat is one problem, but the next problem is what happens inside the animal when eating grain. When an animal is fed grain, especially cows, the animal flesh becomes contaminated with palmitic acid, which may contribute to high cholesterol in humans.[58] The flesh of grain fed animals also has a high ratio of Omega 6 to Omega 3. Animals, including humans, need more Omega 3 over Omega 6. When this ratio is reversed there are many associated health risks, including the increased risk of human insulin resistance and inflammation.[59] Many of us suffer from inflammation. In fact, inflammation is one of the most common symptoms experienced today.

Feeding grain to cows and chickens sounds natural and seems like it should be healthy, but grain is not the ideal diet for an animal that will eventually be slaughtered for human consumption. Instead we should consider grass fed and pasture fed animals. When an animal is allowed to eat pasture and other grasses as its main source of food over grain, the animal fares better and so do we. Grass or pasture fed means the animal flesh becomes the highest quality of animal protein available to humans. Grass fed meat is higher in Omega 3 over 6, and contain four times the amount of Vitamin E and selenium, two nutrients that help protect us from cancer and heart disease.[60]

Grass fed beef is more expensive to buy, and in some places near impossible to find. If grass fed beef and pasture fed eggs (which is not the same as cage free eggs, because cage free could mean grain fed) are not readily available in your grocery store, ask around. Check out your local butcher or local farms and see where your sources of high quality meat and eggs can be found. In the event you cannot find affordable sources of high quality meat and eggs, you may need a different plan for eating meat that will be addressed in your strategies at the end of the chapter.

If we prioritized the quality of our meat by eating meat that contains no growth hormones and made these proteins a part of a plant based diet, then we would not have to give up meat entirely and still achieve better health. Some of the healthiest cultures around the world consume game as their primary source of animal protein. They hunt wild game which means the game is not processed and certainly not injected with growth hormones or implanted with growth implants. Populations from cultures such as Hunza, Equador, Soviet Georgia, and Russians from Caucasus Mountains have a history of good health and longevity with a diet rich in game meat and healthy fat.[61] What if the true culprit in the link between meat consumption and heart disease and cancer had nothing to do with the meat itself and everything to do with the quality of the meat? It would make for an interesting study.

Dr. Weston Price, a well-known dentist of the 20th century, toured the world in search of the nutritional secrets to health and wellness. He discovered those who ate traditional diets of their ancestors that were rich in animal protein and fat, vegetables, fruit and seeds were much healthier over those that ate sugar and processed foods.[62] These people continue to live as humans did before infrastructure, grocery stores and processed food took over our way of living. The people eat very simple diets. Other doctors and scientists discovered similar situations, such as Dr. Emmanuel Cheraskin who found people eating traditional diets rich in protein and void of processed foods had the least amount of health issues.[63]

We need protein. It is the building block of life. Twenty-two amino acids promote muscle development and the nervous system, especially brain health. Without animal proteins we may be deficient in these essential amino acids, Vitamin B12 and iron. Without animal fats we may have trouble absorbing fat-soluble vitamins such as Vitamin A and D. But the poor quality of our meat, mass produced for a profit may be a significant thorn in our side and our health and may be doing more damage than good for the meat eaters in this country. We need to take a stand against hormones in meat; otherwise, we are vulnerable to the consequences of eating poor quality meat. Taking a stand and demanding a better quality of meat can help reduce our toxic load and help restore the traditional benefits of eating meat.

Rule #4: Buy clean animal meat.

What you can do right now:

1. Read the label. Read the label on your meat and dairy products. While a manufacturer does not have to label the use of growth hormones, many manufacturers will label if their products are free of growth hormones. If a company has gone to the trouble to make sure the quality of their products is considerate to your health, they will most likely let their customers know.

2. Eat this instead of that. Organic or range free and hormone free meat is a much, much better choice over meat containing growth hormones, but even better is grass fed beef and pasture fed organic chicken. Cage free eggs are better than conventional eggs, but pasture fed eggs are even better.

3. Think outside the box. If grass fed beef is too expensive, eat chicken, fish and turkey which are easier to digest.

4. Have game time. Consider other sources of clean animal proteins such as game meats including quail, buffalo, bison, venison, elk, boar and fresh caught fish.

5. Make the most of quality. One way to get around the cost of high quality meat is to make the most of it. Buy one quality cut of steak and slice into thin strips for stir-fry, feeding 2-4 people with one cut instead of 2-4 people eating a whole steak each that is not clean. Buy two chicken breasts to feed four, making tacos, burritos, stir-fry, casseroles or soups. Lastly, roast large cuts of meat with the bone, and make soup with the leftover bone and get two meals out of the one cut. Making soup with leftover bones means you get some of the hidden nutrients stored in the animal bone marrow.

6. Refuse to participate. By refusing to buy meats containing hormones, we take a stand against the practices of our government when their actions imply profits over health.

7. Eating out; go without. If you are not sure of the quality of the meat served at a restaurant, it is best to avoid ordering what may be very poor quality meat.

8. Give thanks. Once upon a time, meat was a luxury item even in this country. There are many countries that still have little to no meat. We need to remember and appreciate the availability of quality meat and that we still have a choice between buying meat and dairy with growth hormones and without.

CHAPTER FIVE

How much and how often?

ONCE UPON A time, we farmed in harmony with nature. We lived off the land, eating what was in season and saved meat for Sunday dinner or special occasions. Many families, surviving on their own sustainability, did not slaughter an animal every day to put meat on the table. If we go back even further to an earlier time, before agriculture and farming were the way most people lived, the hunter-gatherer lived off game, which was the cleanest of meats and ate the entire animal believing none should be wasted. Meat was eaten almost all the time. The amount of meat we can safely consume is a controversial subject at best. Much research has been devoted to a vegetarian lifestyle as the path to better health. Yet, the Weston Price foundation, the Paleo Diet, and ancient man refutes the idea that vegetarian is better. This is a long time debate—to eat meat or not to eat meat.

I myself have pondered the debate, read countless books on the subject and initially believed a vegetarian lifestyle was the logical step in my own pursuit of health. The research and the evidence all seemed to make sense. I experienced some initial benefits of becoming vegetarian, such as the detoxification that occurs when going through a fast, and it prompted me to continue. Then about a year into my vegetarian journey my own health suffered a decline. I began experiencing some significant fatigue that I had not experienced before. I decided to take become vegan to help solve the problems that had developed after becoming vegetarian. After all, if giving up some animal products helped, then maybe I should give them all up. But after becoming vegan and giving up all animal products, I then suffered an even further decline in my own health. I went back to the drawing board, did more research and found a balance and unique approach to eating meat and the health issues I experienced went away. Good health is not as straightforward as just whether or not to eat meat.

My own dilemma over eating meat and my personal journey was the inspiration behind much of my personal studies which led to my passion for nutrition and my commitment to help others find the way to optimal health through healthy eating. The decision on whether or not to eat meat is a very heated debate, with popular sources like *The China Study* proving that dietary proteins greatly influenced the growth of cancer tumors.[64] Basically, there is no single diet that works for every single person, but there needs to be more guidance to help you make sense of the information and make decisions appropriate to your health. This chapter will explore health issues surrounding eating meat and how this affects the amount you should be eating.

The question of how much protein the human body needs varies from source to source. The World Health Organization and the National Research Council, claims that only 5-8% of our total caloric intake needs to be protein in order to receive adequate vitamins, minerals and amino acids.[65] Our government recommends a daily allowance of 9-10%, and new and upcoming science as discussed in *The Paleo Diet* recommends up to 20% protein.[66] In actuality, most Americans consume between 15-16%. The problem with 15-16% in the typical American diet is the quality of protein is very poor due to growth hormones at farms, or meats being processed with additives (such as the kind you find in fast food restaurants). Most of the time, when protein is discussed, no one talks about the quality of protein being a direct indicator of how much meat an individual can eat. Let's examine why consideration of the quality is such a vital aspect to the quantity we can eat.

A typical day in the life of an American meat eater may look like this: Egg and sausage biscuit for breakfast, fast food hamburger for lunch, and chicken with pasta for dinner. If this, or something similar, is what you are eating on a typical day, you are leaving yourself wide open to health issues resulting from poor-quality meats possibly processed with additives. We then take poor quality meat and combine it with other poor choices, such as refined white flour bread products that are also filled with additives. If your breakfast was bought in the freezer aisle or your sausage was bought precooked, chances are you are adding even more preservatives and additives. Remember Rule #1: Buy real food.

Fast food meat especially is a real problem for the consumer. Not only does it originate from animals treated with growth hormones, but it is then processed with additive and preservative ingredients such as dimethylpolysiloxane. One of the most harmful additives is found in cured and smoked meats to reduce spoilage. These additives are known as sodium nitrate or nitrites. These additives combine with the protein of the meat to make cancer causing compounds. In fact, consuming these kinds of meat on a regular basis can increase your risk of leukemia, lymphoma and brain cancer.[67] The amount of nitrates in your system matters. According to the *Encyclopedia of Healing Foods* children who eat hot dogs once a week are doubling their chances of developing brain tumors.[68] If your meat is poor in quality and contains additives, then the amount has to be taken into consideration because each time you eat meat containing additives you bring more problems to the table than just growth hormones alone.

How we cook red meat can also influence our health. Studies

show red meat that is grilled to well-done carries a greater risk over browned meat for colon cancer.[69] Meats cooked on high temperatures increase risk of prostate cancer.[70] Charcoaled and smoked meats have even higher cancer risk due to carbon compounds that are created during the smoking, curing or charcoaling process.[71] The hotter the cooking temperature, the more nutrients are cooked away. So not only is charcoal and smoked meats a greater risk for cancer, but also they are more nutritionally depleted from well done meat. Microwaving is technically super high heat cooking. Therefore, microwave cooking will deplete nutrients faster than any other cooking method. Meat needs to be cooked thoroughly. Eating undercooked meat carries its own health risk, such as trichinae, a live parasitic worm found in pork. But microwave cooking, charcoal and smoking needs to be avoided as much as possible.

Many believe becoming vegetarian is the answer, and you cannot refute the many initial benefits to giving up meat. When someone gives up toxic animal proteins, they may feel great for a significant period of time. Giving up meat containing growth hormones and/or additives lessens the toxic load the body is asked to handle and can be very helpful for many people with heavy toxicity or impaired immune systems. Often referred to as detoxification, the reduction of toxins and the toxic load on the body, is very important. Detoxification and cleansing practices that include the elimination of meat have been helpful in many chronic conditions. Many individuals feel so good after detoxification they proclaim themselves vegetarian and give up animal proteins entirely. But giving up *all* animal products for an extended period of time may be more harmful than good. Eventually our bodies will run out of its stores of important nutrients from not only the meats, but the fats that come with them.

Many vegans (individuals who practice eating a diet containing absolutely no animal products) may begin to feel the slow decline of their health after several years, and may not even realize the connection between their health and the missing animal proteins and fats. No other species on the planet is vegan. Even animals thought to be vegetarian, such as gorillas and cattle, meet their complete protein requirements when they eat insects and larvae. Vegetarians that meet their animal protein needs by consuming eggs may have more success with their health over vegans that give up all animal proteins entirely. Health problems such as infertility, bone loss and nervous system complaints may be linked to diets containing little or no animal proteins.[72] Many vegans and vegetarians will turn to supplements to help compensate for missing nutrients we find in animal protein such as B12 and iron. Supplements are a necessary compliment to healthy eating, but should never be a replacement for food nutrients. Many vegans eat soy protein that has been made into meat alternatives, which can also be genetically modified. Soy based meat alternatives are another version of processed food. There is no replacement to the nutrients contained in whole foods and in the benefits of quality animal protein and fat.

Consider some new guidelines. If your regular meat consumption contains growth hormones and includes processed meats such cold cuts, bacon, hot dogs and other meat products or if you consume large quantities of meat at restaurants where you do not know the source, then you may need to follow a conservative guideline of 9–10% protein intake. It would be even more beneficial to drop down to 5% animal protein temporarily while adding more vegetable proteins until you are able to make some changes to the quality of your meat. But, if your animal protein diet is made up of only high quality meats that contain no hormones or antibiotics such as grass fed beef, organic chicken, organic turkey and pasture fed eggs (which is the topic of a later chapter), and you avoid all processed meats, and combine these foods with a plant based diet—then the quality of your meat may allow you to follow up to a 15% daily intake. The only way a higher intake of high quality animal protein will be beneficial to you is when the amount of vegetables you eat totals more than half the amount of meat you consume. If you look closely at studies, it is the reduction of meat in combination with an increase in vegetables that brings about the greatest health benefits such as reducing risk of heart attack, stroke, diabetes and cancer.[73]

If you are not able to find good clean sources of animal protein or you choose not to purchase clean sources, then you still have options to help reduce the health risks associated with low quality meat. The very first is to eliminate meats containing harsh additives such as your fast food meats. Then you need to avoid or reduce high amounts of processed meats such as cold cuts, hot dogs and sausages that contain artificial ingredients and may contain animal remnants. Lastly, you have to reduce or eliminate the amount of meat you consume tainted with growth hormones. This also applies to eggs, where you avoid egg substitutes, and you make sure you buy eggs labeled "cage free" or "pasture fed" eggs as discussed in Chapter Four. In taking such key steps in the management of your meat and egg consumption, you will have helped prevent breast and prostate cancer in your children, reduced your own accelerated aging, and reduced the toxic load of artificial ingredients and the burden those ingredients place on your body.

If you are vegetarian, you may have improved your health greatly by eliminating toxic or inflammatory causing meat. After a time, however, you may suffer from health issues such as low energy, mood issues, irritability, lack of concentration and poor libido because animal proteins and fats also provide for your vitamin B12, iron and amino acid needs. There are many studies to the benefits of a vegetarian lifestyle, but not without adequate protein. Now remember vegetarian means you will eat eggs, and sometimes fish, but not other meats. Adequate amounts of egg and fish can supply your protein needs; it is the vegan who is abstaining from all animal products that may suffer from lack of adequate proteins. Goat dairy and cage free eggs make great sources of protein and should be included in your diet in order to make sure you do not fall victim to health issues associated with a complete lack of animal proteins.

The toxicity of our meat combined with excessive consumption and high heat cooking is a freight train headed for disaster. Common sense tells us so. Not only is hormone free meat a priority, as mentioned earlier, but proteins from grain fed sources should really be eaten minimally if you cannot afford grass fed or pasture raised animal protein. In exchange, other sources of proteins such as legumes need to replace poor quality meat. When we understand the toxicity of our meat, then we can understand how to identify the amount we are supposed to eat. Changes in our health cannot occur unless we first change our understanding of food and how certain types of food, such as meat, will affect us. Animal protein, especially, needs to be understood in a radical new way.

RULE #5: CHANGE YOUR MEAT QUALITY OR EAT LESS OF IT.

What you can do right now:

1. Eliminate meat containing nitrates. Animal proteins such as cold cuts, hot dogs, jerky, sausages and bacon can all contain nitrates. Companies such as Applegate Farms® are making better quality hot dogs, sausages and luncheon meat.

2. Change or reduce. If you cannot change the quality of your meat, then you have to eat less of it.

3. Watch the burn. Limit your consumption of charcoal and smoked meats. Avoid microwave cooking as much as you can.

4. Good portions. A healthy portion of meat is the size of your fist. Anything more than that is too much at one time. When we eat the size of our fist, we don't have to worry about counting grams or ounces in order to be accurate. And each person's fist will vary in size based on their age and weight.

5. Limit red meat and pork. The larger the animal the longer it takes your body to digest the flesh of the animal. Since many of us have a weak digestive system, consider limiting beef and pork. Pork should be avoided as much as possible since they are dirty animals that often eat waste including their own. If you do not want to give up pork entirely, make sure you are eating

organic, cooking to an internal temperature of 160 degrees Fahrenheit, and limiting to once a month.

6. Reduce sugar meats. Pork products like ham and bacon have added sugars in them. So even if you avoid those processed meats containing additives, you have to watch the sugar. Sugar in any food is a problem and is discussed in Chapter Ten.

7. Be a nighttime vegetarian and kick the morning coma. Eating after dark is very hard on the body, and meat takes a very long time to digest. Instead of resting at night, your body is digesting which makes you tired the next morning thinking you need caffeine to get you going. If you find yourself in a situation where eating late is unavoidable, avoiding meat can help your body deal with late night digestion.

8. Take a break. Take a break from eating meat altogether for dinner at least 3-4 times a week. Plan and commit to at least three if not four vegetarian meals a week for dinner. This is not as complicated as you might think with a vegetarian dish containing rice and black beans as your protein base, or a homemade broccoli quiche with eggs for your protein.

9. Keep it complete. Vegetarian meals can include dairy products, eggs or fish. But if your meal is vegan and contains no animal products, then you need to make sure you are consuming a complete protein. A complete protein is made when combining legume (beans) with a grain. An example of this is rice and beans.

10. Keep your money in the bank. Meat is one of the most expensive items in our grocery stores, especially if we are buying high quality meat. Vegetarian options mean less money spent on a meal. Your stomach will thank you, and so will your pocketbook.

11. Watch the bread. Be careful when reducing meat consumption that you do not increase your consumption of wheat or corn. While the subject of grains will be addressed later, your choice

of a vegetarian dinner should never be dominated by refined carbohydrates.

12. Weight loss conscious. If you are watching your weight, not only portions are important but also how you combine your proteins. Animal proteins will digest more efficiently when combined with vegetables and simple starches such as potatoes and squashes. Meat combined with grains is a slow ride through your body.

CHAPTER SIX

Are you a baby cow?

A S A NUTRITIONIST, the question of cow's milk is by far one of the most controversial topics when I speak to groups of people. I often attempt to leave it out of the conversation, but inevitably someone always asks for my opinion on whether or not we should drink cow's milk. The problem is after the question is asked: no one really wants the answer. We are too confused by our love for dairy and our fear of osteoporosis that we are reluctant to consider that milk may not do a body good. This chapter is an in-depth look at milk, whether or not we should consume it, the reasons behind my position and some very manageable strategies to help you make the best health choices surrounding one of man's best loved foods—cow dairy.

The statement "Milk does a body good" is one of many that have convinced Americans to consume vast amounts of milk, but we often fail to understand what milk even is. Milk, in the United States, is the breast milk of a cow designed to grow a baby calf, an already large animal, into a full size cow. Americans drink it in large quantities or eat it in a variety of forms such as cheese and yogurt, but many do not realize there might be a real problem with humans using nature's food designed specifically for the cow.

Why? There are many reasons. First, let's begin with a brief look at the nutrient differences between human and cow's milk in the table below. [74]

	Human breast milk	Cow's breast milk
Protein	7%	19%
Carbohydrate	39%	29%
Fat	54%	52%

If you consider Mother Nature's recommendation for humans, we have a greater need for both fats and carbohydrates over protein in our milk, while cows have a much greater need for protein and significantly less need for carbohydrates. These differences between cow's milk and human milk may be just enough to make cow's milk a problem for humans. In fact, infants who drink infant formula containing milk proteins have a 52% greater chance of developing diabetes later in life.[75] But, it is not just our infants that should be avoiding cow's milk.

The second reason cow's milk can be a real problem for humans, especially adults, is the mature human body does not produce enough enzymes needed to digest milk. After we have completed puberty and finished growing, our biological need for any breast milk is over. Our bodies' production of lactase, the enzyme needed to digest milk, decreases significantly or stops altogether.[76] In many cases when the loss of enzymes to digest breast milk is noticeable enough, we are diagnosed as being lactose intolerant. Then, when cows are treated with antibiotics their milk is even further depleted in enzymes.[77] In summary, cow's milk is different than human breast milk, and becomes very difficult to digest as we age, both from a lack of enzymes in our bodies and from the additives the cow consumes such as hormones and antibiotics. But most people believe that cow's milk is such an important source of calcium that we are not convinced it is dangerous to our health.

The third reason to rethink our dairy consumption is whether or not we truly meet our calcium needs with cow's milk. We have been convinced milk is our only source of dietary calcium and are afraid to eliminate it from our diets. We definitely need calcium for many reasons including the health of our bones. Many of my clients are surprised to find out that, due to our inability to truly break down cow's milk, only 32% of that much needed calcium is actually absorbed.[78] If we absorb so little of the calcium in the milk, cow's milk cannot completely satisfy our calcium needs. Consider other foods such as almonds, carrots, cabbage, and sesame seeds which contain more useable calcium to provide you with the added calcium you need. Consuming foods containing more useable calcium means more of it is absorbed, and the body benefits much more.

The next reason to examine cow's milk is growth hormones. Growth hormones in milk pose serious health risks. They find their way into most of the milk produced in this country. If a milk product is hormone-free, it is labeled as such. Growth hormones in dairy, like in meat, increase farmers' and manufacturers' production at your expense. As discussed in Chapter Four, when fed indirectly to children through meat and dairy, growth hormones have been linked to early onset puberty and associated with increased risk of breast and prostate cancer. Studies have shown the growth hormones in milk to pose a greater risk of these cancers, especially prostate cancer.[79]

The next major problem with cow's milk is pasteurization. Pasteurization is basically heating the milk to slow down the spoilage rate and reduce, not eliminate the potential number of pathogens in the milk. But this is done at the expense of necessary amino acids that help break down the excess proteins and other necessary vitamins and minerals such as C, B12, calcium, magnesium and potassium.[80] Even now, a number of chronic conditions like Crohn's disease are being linked to pasteurized cow's milk.[81]

It would all be worth it if we could guarantee that pasteurization protects us against contaminated milk, but it does not. In 1985 an outbreak of salmonella occurred in pasteurized milk, effecting 14,000 people in the state of Indiana[82] and proving that pasteurization is not failsafe. And several outbreaks of Listeriosis have been linked to pasteurized dairy products.[83] According to the Center for Disease Control Prevention, the bacteria Yersinia enterocolitica was found in pasteurized Grade A milk and ice cream in Pennsylvania as recently as July 2011. Of the sixteen people affected, seven were sent to the hospital and three were admitted into an intensive care unit. Yersinia enterocolitica is not typically seen in pasteurized milk and milk products, samples of Grade A milk, yet the bacteria was able to penetrate pasteurization's protection along with various other pathogens throughout the years. This leads us to question whether pasteurization truly protects us.

If pasteurization does not fully protect us against pathogens while reducing the milk's nutritional value and our ability to digest an already complicated to digest food, then the alternative would seem to be unpasteurized milk, also known as raw milk. Weston Price foundation promotes the consumption of raw dairy, stating cultures eating traditional diets that include raw (unpasteurized) whole milk and other raw dairy products proved themselves to be healthier overall. Supporters of this idea have led a movement back to consuming raw milk. However, this has also led to the study of raw milk and with it some unexpected results.

In a recent Japanese study, in an attempt to examine the true risk surrounding the consumption of raw milk, researchers discovered that an antibiotic-resistant strain of bacteria, Klebsiella pneumonia, existed in both raw and pasteurized milk.[84] This resistant strain was also found in both conventional and organic farms. Widespread contamination of drug-resistant Klebsiella pneumonia in the dairy industry could be a grave threat to farmers and consumers of pasteurized milk, both conventional and organic, as well as raw, unpasteurized milk. While organic farms may protect consumers from the use of growth hormones and antibiotics, the consumer can still be at risk for resistant bacteria multiplying in the dairy cow population around the world. While this study did not necessarily prove that raw milk was more vulnerable to bacteria over pasteurized milk, it did reveal another troubling aspect to the consumption of dairy in general—the drug-resistant bacteria.

In other areas, there is great concern over the handling of raw milk. In Tunisia, where bovine tuberculosis is still a chronic condition and where the consumption of raw milk is prevalent, studies indicate raw milk drinkers are at greater risk for infection from cow's testing positive for bacteria M. bovis.[85] In other rural places around the world where the handling of raw, pasteurized or boiled milk may be compromised, the safety of dairy products altogether is questionable. In Mali, Africa where dairy products are a staple, a 2004 study proved both raw and pasteurized dairy to be a source of toxic bacteria. In this case, raw milk was not the true culprit; in fact researchers stated individuals consuming pasteurized milk were four times as likely to contract food related toxic infections.[86] And in areas of Poland, where tick borne encephalitis is prevalent, all raw milk was contaminated anywhere from 10-22% of the time with the tick borne encephalitis virus that has been linked to meningitis in approximately 50% of cases. Tick borne encephalitis virus may affect the nervous system resulting in a potentially serious infection.[87] Geographic areas where animals are more susceptible to tick bites require more diligence in the handling of raw milk, and certainly research suggests that these geographic areas should pasteurize their milk to reduce the risk of contamination.

The safety of raw milk largely depends on the handling conditions and temperature control efforts that include keeping milk at specific cold temperatures. However, similar to the evolution of drug resistant bacteria, there are species of bacteria that are proving to be cold resistant.[88] Maybe Mother Nature is trying to tell us something? Maybe milk should go straight from its mother to its young, and any variation of this risks consequence.

Many of our health issues with milk begin very young. Infants who drink infant formula containing cow's milk proteins have a 52% greater chance of developing diabetes later in life.[89] From infancy, many children develop an allergy to cow's milk protein. Approximately 26% of children have an allergy to milk contributing to gastrointestinal issues, skin issues such as eczema, respiratory issues and even anaphylactic shock which can sometimes result in death.[90] Another significant problem associated with consuming cow dairy during childhood is constipation. Over 15% of children see their pediatrician for constipation alone, and the leading cause in most of these cases is cow's dairy.[91] And constipation is not an affliction reserved for the young. Many adults also suffer from a variety of colon issues, with colon cancer being a prevalent and epidemic problem in this country. Concerns with cow's milk also means that products made from cow's milk such as butter, yogurt, and cheese can all carry similar health issues. Let's take a bigger look at one of man's favorite dairy product, cheese.

Cheese is a favorite food around the world, but many of us have no idea how cheese is made. Cheese is milk that has been acidified (soured) and then a particular ingredient is added to change the chemistry of the milk making it into different flavors and consistencies. These ingredients will curdle the sour milk and or set the cheese into a rubbery gel. A number of different agents are used such as vinegar, lemon juice, vegetable sources called vegetable rennet (made from fungus) or enzymes. Other cheeses are often made with a different substance entirely called animal rennet.

Animal rennet is pieces of cut up baby cow stomach, specifically the inner mucosa of the fourth stomach of a calf. It is cleaned and dried and added to saltwater where vinegar or other ingredients are added. This animal rennet mixture is added to the soured milk. After a period of time, the milk is filtered and cheese results salt is used to help preserve the cheese. Cheese is also very high in casein, a milk protein. Casein is very difficult to digest for anyone who has any digestive issue.

Many of us are unwilling to give up dairy completely, at least not the cheese part. So, if you are unwilling to give up cheese completely, you should have some strategies for making the best possible choices. Consider easier to digest cheeses such as organic raw cheeses, organic pasteurized cheeses, and cheese made with vegetable rennet or water bathed cheeses. Raw cheese contains all the enzymes to help break the milk proteins down because it has not been pasteurized, but be sure to buy organic when dealing in raw to minimize risk factors. Cheese made with vegetable rennet is free of animal rennet. Or you can consider goat cheese made from goat milk.

Goat products are an important alternative to cow's milk products, especially for growing and developing children. Goat milk has been proven to be easier to digest, often resolves gastrointestinal distress, asthma and eczema.[92] Even though there is doubt surrounding goat milk as a complete replacement for cow's milk for those allergic, evidence suggests goat milk can be considered an alternative to cow's milk.[93]

During a child's development, especially prior to and during puberty, calcium needs may not be met through other food sources alone. Goat's milk supplies the needed calcium and nutrients without the complicated proteins and compromised digestibility. Studies show children that consume goat's milk instead of cow's milk experience greater growth, better height and weight and better overall nutrient content to their blood.[94] Strategies such as changing to goat milk are one of many to help us improve our health when it comes to dairy.

RULE #6: CHOOSE YOUR DAIRY PRODUCTS WISELY.

What you can do right now:

1. Go organic and go whole. If you are going to drink milk at least switch to organic *whole* milk. Yes, whole milk so the fat can help break down the protein. And organic, so that you at least eliminate the hormones, antibiotics and pesticides used in conventional dairy farms.

2. Reach for the almond milk. Try almond milk as an alternative

to cow's milk. There are a lot of different non-dairy milks such as rice milk, hemp milk, soy milk and coconut milk. Rich in protein, calcium and healthy fats, unsweetened almond milk is the best choice of the alternative milks.

3. Eat this, not that. Consume organic, pasture fed or grass fed butter over conventional butter. And if you cannot buy pasture fed or grass fed butter, real butter is still a better choice over margarine. Since many toxins found in dairy are located in the milk water, as opposed to the milk fat, butter is less problematic for most people but still should be of the highest quality. Regular butter is fine in moderation, but organic is even better, and organic pasture fed or grass fed is best. Eating real butter over margarine reduces the health risks associated with synthetic food products, and when your butter is organic you avoid health risks associated with pesticides and hormones that result from conventional farming and manufacturing.

4. Know your cheese. Read your labels and know which cheeses are made with animal rennet and which ones are not. Avoid cheese that is made with animal rennet, the cut up stomach lining of cow. Switch to easier to digest cheeses that are made with vegetable rennet. Groceries stores such as Whole Foods Market will label their cheese as being made with vegetable rennet or animal rennet. Or switch to cheese that is kneaded or washed in warm water which will lower the acidity of the cheese such as mozzarella, provolone, Edam, Gouda and Colby cheese. Mozzarella is the only cheese that can be found packaged in water, but it is the processing and not the packaging that is crucial.

5. Fermented and plain. Consume fermented dairy such as plain yogurt, which may allow more effective digestion of the lactase and casein since fermentation predigests the milk. Avoiding sugar and sweetener laced yogurts is a much better choice for your immune system. Yogurt is counter-productive to

our health when sugar is added or, worse yet, when yogurt is made with aspartame or food dyes. Organic plain yogurt (with NO sugar or sweeteners) is more easily tolerated by the digestive system. If eating plain yogurt makes your face pucker, try adding raw honey or pure maple syrup to a plain yogurt and avoid the damaging sugars added to the yogurt prior to packaging.

6. Keep the sugar stuff clean. Many of us like our ice cream. Ice cream is dairy combined with sugar. This combination can be a real problem for many people, because one, the combination of sugar and dairy proteins is very difficult to digest and two, artificial ingredients such as polysorbate 80 brings unwanted chemicals into our body. Sugar is often genetically modified. Ice cream should be organic both for the milk quality and sugar quality to minimize the hurt.

7. Avoid combining dairy and wheat. Since both cow dairy and wheat often stimulate the body in an unhealthy manner, avoid combining the two foods at one sitting to reduce the shock on the body. An example of this, if you are going to have ice cream, first make sure it is high quality such as organic made from real cream, but then have it in a dish, not a cone.

8. Try goat instead. Goat milk is a closer to human breast milk than cow's milk. Goat milk is more easily tolerated, is easier to digest and is a better choice for developing children. Goat milk has been made into a variety of foods such as butter, yogurt, kefir and both soft and hard cheeses.

CHAPTER SEVEN

My, what small teeth you have.

OST PEOPLE BELIEVE that fish is a take it or leave it food. Either you like seafood or you don't. What if I told you that fish is literally responsible for better brains? It is true. One of my favorite nutritional stories is related to fish. Scientists discovered that the evolution and growth of the human brain is now credited to the introduction of seafood into our diets. Basically they found that groups of people that lived closer to seashores and added fish and other seafood to their diet increased the gray matter of their brains. When the gray matter increased, so did human intelligence. Fossil studies indicate this change in the cerebral cortex happened only to humans that added seafood to their diet; and as a result added key nutrients such as EPA (eicosapentaenoic acid) and DHA (docosahexaenoic acid). EPA and DHA are the two most digestible forms of Omega 3, an essential fatty acid. These particular nutrients are the ones that have a positive effect on the brain.[95] This chapter discusses the importance of fish, and how to purchase and consume it safely.

Fish is also one of the most important foods in the fight against cardiovascular disease and may lower risk against breast cancer, prostate, colon and lung cancer. Fish even provides health benefits for conditions such as asthma, depression, high blood pressure and inflammatory conditions such as arthritis.[96] Fish has quite a resume in the fight for our health. All fish and shellfish contain Omega 3, but some fish have higher and more beneficial levels than others. The highest concentrations of Omega 3 are found in salmon, mackerel, tuna, whitefish and herring.[97] Bass, mussels and oysters, rainbow trout, and swordfish come in second in their Omega 3 content. Eating fish and shellfish containing Omega 3 means we are taking care of our brains, our hearts and our intestinal track.

The negative effect to eating seafood is the growing concern over mercury and other toxins that fill our oceans and have contaminated our fish. It is very sad that such an important food in the evolution of humans as a species has now fallen prey to our ignorant destruction of their home and our waters. As a result, we now have to protect ourselves against the growing toxicity of our waters and seafood. Fresh water fish are often contaminated with pesticides, and large ocean fish are often contaminated with mercury and other toxins, and have a greater chance of toxins due to their size. The most prevalent of toxins include mercury, PCBs, chlorade, dioxins, and DDT.[98] And recently we need to be afraid of genetically modified fish such as salmon.

We need to eat fish, at least twice a week. But how do we do this safely, keeping in mind our health and the environment? One way is to eat small fish. Small fish such as herring, sardines, and anchovies can have fewer toxins over larger fish.[99] The reason they have less toxins, is all living animals store many of their toxins in the fat tissue, and the smaller the fish, the less fat they have on their bodies. Another good way to each fish is to eat fish that is not endangered. Mackerel is not endangered, and high in useable calcium when canned, whereas

Bluefin and Bigeye tuna are both endangered. Tuna is also a very large fish and considered high in mercury. You can also consider buying local and line caught, or from organic farms which means we are getting a fresher fish that is more environmentally sound, and good for our health.

The way we cook fish is also important. Cooking fish on a rack or grill will also reduce toxic exposure since the fat storing toxins will drip off during the cooking process. Lastly, cooking side dishes with turmeric may help carry toxins like mercury out of the body and in doing so improves the nutritional value of this great food. We need the nutritional value of these foods in our diet, especially salmon.

Salmon could be the most important fish to eat. Salmon is rich in nutrients such as protein, Vitamin B12, selenium, potassium, niacin and phosphorus. A three ounce serving contains approximately 1,000mg of EPA and 725 mg of DHA.[100] Wild Alaskan salmon is one of the safest salmon as well as organic farmed salmon. Fish such as tuna and halibut have much more risk of mercury and other toxins due to their size and age, both contributing to a greater storage of toxins in their body. Large fish such as tuna should be consumed no more than once a month, and when someone has a health crisis, such as mercury toxicity, tuna and other large fish should not be eaten at all.

Hopefully we can continue to learn how to eat fish safely, but the rapid destruction of our oceans needs to be stopped in order to ensure that our grandchildren will even have fish to eat. Protecting our oceans is not just for the benefit of seafood on our plate, but the continued supply of oxygen, energy and nutrients that help keep this planet running smoothly. Organizations, such as Greenpeace International, are working towards making sure 40% of our oceans are made into protected reserves just like our national parks protect our lands. This strategy is one of the few ways we can ensure the quality of our seafood and our planet.

Rule #7: Eat small fish at least twice a week.

What you can do right now:

1. Eat small. The smaller the fish, the less likely it is to have accumulated years of toxins and this may reduce your risk of toxic exposure. Small fish such as herring, sardines and anchovies are rich in Omega 3 and are safe to eat.

2. Eat often. Fish and some shellfish such as mussels contain important nutrients to help protect us against heart disease, high blood pressure, certain cancers and most of all provide important nutrients for our brain. At least once a week, seafood should be on your menu.

3. Think pink. Salmon is one of the most important fish we can eat. If you cannot afford salmon filet, canned salmon is an affordable and nutrient rich alternative.

4. Keep the flavor. Salmon is often overcooked and this can dry the fish and take some of the flavor with it. Dry fish is not nearly as tasty as moist and juicy fish. Carefully cook salmon and check often with a thermometer to make sure you cook thoroughly but do not overcook.

5. Buy local or organic. Local fish is often less expensive and will carry more nutrients due to the freshness. Organic fish farms such as salmon and tilapia cause less pollution than regular fish farms. Buying organic farmed tilapia means a better quality of a fish that can otherwise bottom feed in certain conditions. Conventional salmon are often given food dyes either indirectly in their fish food or directly coloring the fish to sell.

6. Limit eating bottom feeders. Full-time bottom feeders such as crab, lobster, catfish, halibut, snails, clams, bluefish, flounder, sole, grouper, carp, and shrimp are more likely to consume toxic sediment that fall to the bottom of the ocean floor. Some bottom feeders have a plant based diet, but others are eating

other bottom feeders. All in all, bottom feeders are more likely to carry a greater toxic load.

7. Bake on a rack. Toxins are most likely stored in fat. Cooking larger fish on a grill or rack and allowing the fat to drip off the fish means the toxins have a chance to drip off as well.

8. Cook with turmeric and cilantro. Turmeric is the bright yellow and flavorless spice used in Indian cooking. This spice is also known for its ability to help with toxins in the body. Heavy metals in particular, such as mercury, can be moved through the body more efficiently when eating turmeric. Make a side dish to your fish or seafood with yellow rice made from Jasmine rice and turmeric. Add some diced cilantro, which also has properties for helping move mercury out of the body.

9. Eat canned mackerel or salmon. If fresh fish is too expensive for you, consider canned mackerel or salmon, which is inexpensive and still rich in Omega 3 and even calcium from the small bones mixed in with the fish.

10. Frequent the Marine Conservation Society. The Marine Conservation Society located at www.mcsuk.org provides updated information on what fish is safe to eat and what fish is not in their "Good Fish Guide". At this time, organic farmed salmon is safe to eat, whereas general stocks of Atlantic salmon are not recommended. American lobster is not recommended, but mussels are safe. Pacific cod is recommended over much of the Atlantic cod.

11. Support Greenpeace International's plan for marine reserves. At http://www.greenpeace.org/international/en/campaigns/oceans/marine-reserves/ you can find all kinds of wonderful information about the importance of protecting our oceans. We need to do this for our planet.

PART III

Let's get real about starches, sweets and fats.

"The part can never be well unless the whole is well."
—Plato

CHAPTER EIGHT

Gluten, gluten and more gluten.

M Y GRANDMOTHER CAME to this country from Italy. The love of Italian food is in my blood, and that's a lot of pasta. In spite of how wonderfully breads and pastas taste, there are some significant health issues related to the over consumption of food products made with refined carbohydrates like white flour. These refined carbohydrates become even more difficult to digest when we add white sugar, high fructose corn syrup and various kinds of oils such as transfat. In this country we have over processed our grains, added stabilizers and preservatives until the body can no longer handle the assault and the grain itself is now a real problem in our health. The result is an overwhelming reduction of the nutritional benefits of wheat and the interference with the absorption of other nutrients.

I continue to be amazed how many of my clients feel so much better when they eliminate refined carbohydrates from their diets. Complete elimination of gluten (the protein within the wheat grain) altogether may be necessary for some of you, but many of you may not have to go that far. This chapter will help you understand the many health problems related to over consuming refined carbohydrates that contain gluten, a troublesome protein found in wheat and other grains, and what to do about it.

Most of us eat too many foods made with refined carbohydrates in relation to the amount of whole foods we eat, especially fruits and vegetables. Many of these refined carbohydrates are processed and in this country, tend to also contain synthetic, or man-made, ingredients to help preserve and make shelf worthy this already difficult to digest food. White flour is made into hundreds of different foods from it like breads, muffins, cereals, cookies, crackers, snack cakes, and pasta to name a few.

Take a minute and think about what you ate yesterday for breakfast, snacks, lunch and dinner. Probably most of you had some version of wheat or white flour each time you ate—a bagel or muffin for breakfast, some crackers with cheese for snack, sandwich for lunch, and pasta or bread with dinner. We can literally spend an entire day eating very little but processed foods made with wheat and think we have eaten a variety all day. The truth is, if we primarily fill our day with processed foods, the overwhelming majority of our consumption is most likely only three or four ingredients in an entire day: white flour, white sugar (or high fructose corn syrup,) vegetable oil and maybe dairy. Consuming so little variety by the end of the day leaves our nutritional savings account empty. Like our current economic debt, we have borrowed against our health for far too long. And now the debt is calling.

For many of us it begins with a protein called gluten. Gluten is contained in grains, specifically wheat, spelt, kamut, rye, barley, and triticale. Foods high in gluten are incredibly complicated for the body to digest. These grains have evolved over time, and our digestive systems have evolved over time, elevating our sensitivity. When we struggle digesting this food we can find ourselves faced with slower metabolism, bloating, poor protein absorption and poor absorption of B vitamins. Over 100 different symptoms, including headaches and digestive issues, and conditions such as asthma, cancers and even miscarriages have been linked to the consumption of gluten.[101] We simply cannot feel better if we do not address our excessive gluten consumption.

In simple terms, when eating processed foods, or eating food that contains these grains, the body may react as if invaded by a microbe instead of nourishing food. We can call this non celiac gluten sensitivity. For some of us, our body is literally making antibodies to this grain treating it as a toxin. For some of us, due to a variety of different reasons we may not break down gluten. These undigested molecules can sometimes enter the bloodstream and bind to opiate receptors in the brain causing a host of issues including food addictions. For some, the reaction is much more severe where the body attacks itself resulting in an autoimmune disease called celiac. While only a percentage of individuals have celiac, these numbers are growing. And an even greater percentage of people have non-celiac gluten sensitivity—in fact it is estimated that about 90 million Americans have some version of gluten sensitivity.[102] But the idea of giving up wheat for many is a horrific idea. They feel they are giving up "everything" they currently eat.

If your diet primarily consists of white flour processed foods, and you are addicted to refined carbohydrates, you may be leaking undigested food particles into your blood stream causing other food sensitivities. You are at tremendous health risk if you do not pay attention to the warning sign your addiction is. The number of people in this country diagnosed with celiac is growing as the processing of food increases.[103] Gluten sensitivity hardly exists in underdeveloped areas. Developed countries manufacture and consume more processed food than underdeveloped areas, and we use wheat more than any other grain. We have a problem. Our history with this grain has led us down a path of illness and disease, and we have to face the consequences.

Wheat originated in the Middle East approximately 10,000 years ago.[104] It was originally prepared by mixing the whole grain with water, or grinding the whole grain and then mixing it with water. Today's milling process extracts the bran from the grain, removing approximately 72% of the grain and taking about half the nutrients with it. What we have left is softer, whiter and more appealing to the palate,—but at the expense of our health.[105]

Removing nutrients, while processing wheat, increases our risk for health issues. When we eat this refined version of wheat, where 72% of the grain is removed, the body suffers from poor absorption, poor metabolism and will be missing vitamins and minerals.[106] The consequences are not just the missing nutrients, but all the health issues that are the result of a eating a poorly made food. Zinc, a prime example, is removed during milling. Thus, it can no longer help remove lead and cadium from the grain during digestion. This, in turn, allows a toxic buildup of both lead and cadium in the body.[107] When the body is depleted in zinc there may be digestive issues, skin issues and fertility issues. Zinc and other nutrient loss, especially loss of B vitamins is what prompted the "enrichment" of white flour products. B vitamins are essential to our good health, but it is not enough to enrich the food with these additional nutrients. The human body will always deal with whole food nutrients better than enrichment of the nutrients back into the food.

We cannot just eat the right nutrients, our bodies have to be able to absorb the nutrients we eat. When we don't absorb properly, it is like we never ate those nutrients at all. When eating gluten we may improperly absorb B vitamins and Vitamin D.[108] All B vitamins are necessary for stress relief, energy and proper assimilation of proteins. When B vitamins are depleted, the body is stressed. Vitamin D is fundamental to overall life. If we do not have enough Vitamin D, then it does not matter how much calcium we consume; we may still be in jeopardy of bone loss. Vitamin D also helps our immune system against environmental allergies, food sensitivities and upper respiratory infections.

Absorption issues are not the only concern with autoimmune disease on the rise. Gluten is now being linked to symptoms in autoimmune diseases, not just celiac, and also rheumatoid arthritis, hypothyroidism, multiple sclerosis and juvenile diabetes.[109] Many of my own clients experience a great deal of relief from their arthritis symptoms when following a low-inflammatory diet that includes the elimination of high inflammatory foods that contain gluten. Many children and teens that I have helped were pre-diabetic and have shown tremendous improvement in their health with a diet that includes the elimination of gluten. Many other clients who eliminate gluten improve emotional and mental health issues. Since symptoms will often diminish with a gluten free diet, gluten is currently being researched in brain conditions such as schizophrenia.[110]

While many people experience these and other great improvements in their health with the elimination of gluten, there are those that fail to experience results because they only address gluten elimination and not their overall diet. The success of a gluten free diet is also dependent on improving your overall diet. If you change the pretzel to a gluten free pretzel and still do not eat fruits and vegetables, you may still suffer symptoms associated with the inability to process refined carbohydrates, or you may continue to suffer from the breakdown in your digestive system or you may continue to feed pathogens and fungus in the body. Repair on the body may still need to be addressed.

Removing gluten will only remove any problems you might be experiencing with gluten itself, such as mood and behavioral issues, digestive issues and brain fog, but will not bring total relief if you are experiencing problems with refined or simple carbohydrates in general, such as yeast overgrowth in the body. Consequently, if you do not increase the amounts of whole, quality fruits and vegetables with high quality animal proteins that have not been cured or processed with refined carbohydrates, you will not feel better. If many of us had a plant based diet to begin with combined with whole grains and quality animal proteins in moderation, we may have avoided the challenges with gluten altogether. Therefore, it becomes absolutely crucial to not only reduce or eliminate the gluten, depending on your health, but to increase plant based foods until they make up the bulk of your diet. Celiac requires not only the complete removal of gluten from your diet, but also the use of cookware and kitchen appliances, such as toasters and utensils, that have never come in contact with gluten. Gluten sensitivity on the other hand, can be addressed through reduction or elimination. If you are ready to reduce or eliminate gluten, you will need some strategies.

RULE #8: RETHINK GLUTEN, THEN REDUCE OR ELIMINATE IT FROM YOUR DAILY DIET.

What can you do right now:

1. Reduce or eliminate gluten. If you want to eliminate it slowly, take each of the following strategies in order as baby steps. To eliminate gluten quickly, use the strategies below to help know what foods or types of foods to consider and avoid. If you decide to keep gluten in your diet, remember the quality and the quantity will go a long way to reducing symptoms associated with the over consumption of simple carbohydrates or high inflammatory food. At the end of the day, gluten should be looked at as an exception to our daily diet, and not a staple. Balance and moderation is essential if you choose to consume gluten. All of the following strategies are worth experimenting with to find the right balance of gluten, simple carbohydrates, animal protein and, most importantly, whole fruits and vegetables to improve your health.

2. Run from bleached flour. This is your first step to reduce or gradually eliminate gluten from your diet. Unless the label says "unbleached white flour" chances are the white flour is white because it is bleached using benzoyl peroxide or chlorine gas. Bleaching, in and of itself does not change the nutritional value significantly, since white flour has little value anyway, but it is another processing step we can

do without. Stop and think about it. Why would you eat something that has been bleached?

3. Follow Rule #1– Eat real food. Many processed foods made with flour use preservatives (such as calcium propionate, sorbic acid, cellulose gum,) dough conditioners (such as fumaric acid, sodium metabisulfite, and DATEM) and other stabilizers to extend the shelf life of these products. Extended shelf life ultimately means extended shelf life inside your body as well, making digestion harder on your body. If we are going to eat a complicated food, shouldn't we make sure it does not have long term shelf life, but can be broken down in a day or two? Feel bloated or have heartburn? Eating foods that are designed for extended shelf life may be why.

4. Avoid white flour. The next step is to avoid eating even unbleached flour products on a daily basis. Switch to whole grains or sprouted wheat to continue the transition to improve the quality of your gluten.

5. Watch the combo. Make sure if you do eat gluten, especially white flour products, that you avoid combining it with animal protein. By avoiding these combinations, you ask your digestive system to handle a less complicated load. If you are trying to lose weight avoiding animal flesh (hard to digest) with gluten (hard to digest) may make your metabolic system run more efficiently.

6. Eat gluten sparingly. Next is to begin to reduce your gluten intake. Many of us could not go a whole day without eating some version of wheat even though many of us should be avoiding this food altogether. Begin with reducing daily consumption down to once a day, and then begin eliminating consuming it on a daily basis and reduce consumption down to once a week.

7. Try 90 day elimination. The next step is to take the elimination challenge. Gluten is really a very problematic food, and one

sure way of understanding the truth about this food on your own body is to eliminate it for 90 consecutive days. It takes approximately 21 days to remove a food completely from our digestive system, and 90 days to remove the food particles from our bloodstream. The only true elimination program is 90 day elimination. If you choose to reintroduce gluten after the 90-day elimination, start slowly with high quality gluten foods, keeping strategies 2 and 4 in mind. See how your body reacts and adjust quantities and combinations as necessary, keeping strategies 5 and 6 in mind. Remember that strategies 3 and 8-10 should become, if they haven't already, consistent or habitual. As you continue to reintroduce gluten in its various forms, you will gain great knowledge of how to reach your most beneficial balance of gluten, refined carbohydrates, whole fruits and vegetables and animal proteins.

8. Watch the replacement. It is not in your health's best interest to replace a white flour or wheat flour product with a gluten-free simple carbohydrate every time. Individuals with gluten issues most often have developed less drastic, but none the less, problematic issues with other simple carbohydrates. Replacing a major offending food with a less offending food is still eating an offending food. Replace the gluten with a healthy source of protein, or a fruit or vegetable. For example, if you are removing the pretzels or crackers for a snack, try replacing with a handful of raw almonds and a piece of fruit, instead of trying to find which gluten free pretzel, cracker or cookie taste the most like the problem food you were previously eating. If it is meal time, try replacing the starch portion on your plate with a baked acorn squash drizzled with pure maple syrup, a great compliment to chicken or beef. Pasta primavera or pasta with meat sauce can become stuffed bell peppers with ground meat, onion, carrot, fennel, and tomato sauce over the top. Recipes with the Paleo diet in mind are a great resource for more ideas of how to make meals that are refined carbohydrate free.

9. Almond replacements. If you are going to eat a muffin or a pancake, try some made with almond meal instead of any grain flour. While gluten free flours are a good choice, almond meal means you are using a protein instead of a grain that contains healthy fat and a good source of calcium.

10. Watch the corn. Corn is not a replacement staple for wheat. And the next chapter will tell you why.

CHAPTER NINE

Danger: Corn

$\mathcal{I}$ BEGAN TO FURTHER research corn when my son's mouth began swelling and blistering whenever he ate anything with corn in it, including trace amounts found in ingredients like baking powder or vanilla extract. Since the area around his mouth would swell and blister, it became pretty important to find out all the foods corn is in and all the ingredient names where corn is the source, like dextrose. Suddenly I was keenly aware of just how much packaged food contains some form of this grain from corn sugars to corn starch. Researching corn is difficult. The idea that all corn might be bad for you is a new idea, and not many health care professionals focus on eliminating corn from the diet. High fructose corn syrup is a very well-known and well researched problem, and now GMO's are making corn gain more attention, but the other ideas I present in this chapter are not common knowledge. The ideas in this chapter are radical, but so many of my clients that are willing to take that extra step of eliminating corn often find more emotional stability and less digestive issues. Chapter Three discussed the genetic modification of corn, but this chapter will help you take your diet and health to the next level by focusing on health issues associated ingredients like high fructose corn syrup, corn oil and corn itself.

Corn as a whole food has been a staple crop in the United States since its beginning. Until food manufacturing became so prevalent, it was eaten in its whole form or ground into flour. Now, it has become one of the most processed of all our foods. So many processed foods contain some form of processed corn that like processed wheat, it is becoming an overwhelming factor in many of our health concerns. For example, from a manufacturer's view, foods must have added sweeteners, like high fructose corn syrup, to make them more palatable and additives/preservatives to increase their consumer pool by allowing time for shipping and shelf-sitting in stores and pantries. High fructose corn syrup accounts for approximately 45% of added sweeteners.[111] Other corn ingredients used by most manufacturers include corn starch, corn syrup, and corn meal. These are obviously made from corn, but how many of the foods you eat also contain other not so recognizable forms of corn like dextrose, maltodextrin, monodiglycerides, diglycerides, and monosodium glutamate. The amounts of all these forms of corn added to the amount of whole corn that we eat are becoming increasingly dangerous to our health.

High fructose corn syrup is a combination of glucose and fructose, both derived in a lab. It is very inexpensive (half the price of sugar), has longer shelf life, is reported to enhance the flavor of processed foods and is easier to use from a manufacturer's standpoint.[112] The health issues associated with high fructose corn syrup are not something to take lightly. Consuming high fructose corn syrup (HFCS) is associated with obesity (a huge epidemic in this country), metabolic syndrome (a group of risk factors for cardiac disease and diabetes), insulin resistance, and high cholesterol,[113] increased risk of heart disease, elevated triglycerides, increased risk of cancer, irritable bowel syndrome and functional bowel disease.[114] Having some of these issues can even lead to further health problems. For example, high levels of triglycerides often occur with high uric acid, which is a contributing factor in gout and heart disease.[115]

Much recent press has been paid to the growing problem of obesity in this country, but high fructose corn syrup is still a staple ingredient without even a warning label. Obesity has its own set of concerns such as diabetes, sleep disorders, and glucose intolerance.[116] There was a time when cigarette packs did not contain a warning label, but times did change. Maybe we can hope for the same. Warning: High fructose corn syrup may be dangerous to your health, causing weight gain, obesity, increased risk of cancer, heart disease, bowel disease and contributing to gout and a list of other stuff to lengthy to print.

Some studies are trying to dispute the connection between high fructose corn syrup and obesity in spite of the evidence suggesting the direct correlation between high fructose corn syrup and weight gain.[117] If science proves that eating high fructose corn syrup does not make you gain weight directly, there is still a strong possibility that high fructose corn syrup shuts down appetite control centers.[118] This means it may not put the pounds on, but it may keep you from knowing when to stop eating. High fructose corn syrup is also an ingredient in many junk foods, in many processed and simple carbohydrates that contribute to weight gain. There may even been an indication that high fructose corn syrup is metabolized into fat by the liver.[119] There really is no way around the fact that high fructose corn syrup is a problem for the body and maybe one of the more serious ingredients contributing to our demise.

Unfortunately, high fructose corn syrup is not the only problem food derived from corn. Corn oil is a commonly, refined oil used in cooking that is high in polyunsaturated Omega 6. Omega 6 has now been linked to inflammation. And inflammation is now being linked to cancer.[120] When measured against canola oil for its effect on inflammation and the potential risk for cancer, corn oil, even in the smallest amounts, increases inflammation more than canola oil,[121] which means corn oil carries a greater risk for cancer over canola oil.

Both are genetically modified and both should be avoided. One study compared the effects of corn to butter and coconut oil, and still corn oil was more damaging.[122] The most interesting study had participants consume corn oil as their only source of dietary fat and eliminating all other forms of fat, including animal fat. Their result was an increased death rate by 364% over participants remaining on a diet of saturated fats.[123] If corn oil is even harder on the body than saturated fats, we should probably avoid it.

Turning corn into oils and sugars isn't the only reason corn is a problem food, there is a significant problem with the grain itself, especially for agricultural practices, animal feed production, as well as human consumption, and it is the aflatoxin, a particular form of mycotoxin, a toxic fungus that contaminates certain crops.[124] Mycotoxins are found in peanuts, corn, cotton, and sugar. Mycotoxins are harmful to humans, and aflatoxin is particularly harmful. Aflatoxins are now linked to cancer.[125] Aflatoxin contamination is such a large problem that farmers and agricultural science organizations are looking at different insects and climate conditions to determine possible causes of and solutions to aflatoxin contamination.[126]

Research is also being done to see if natural substances such as clay can bind the aflatoxins before they reach animal feed or human consumption.[127] But until then? Excessive contamination of aflatoxins can cause liver failure. Aflatoxins are dangerous and considered one of the most powerful natural carcinogens. Can we really be sure that we are kept from being exposed to high levels? The only true way to limit your exposure is to limit your own consumption.

Corn was a crop this country was founded on, from Native Americans to Pilgrims. In today's America, we have genetically modified corn. We turn corn into high fructose corn syrup, and we refine corn into corn oil taking this crop far from the sweet goodness it used to be. As you continue this journey for your health, it is important to be aware of the negative influence of this crop in spite of the fact that there is not a lot of research against eating corn. I believe in the next five to ten years more and more research will be available on the harm of this crop. In the meantime, I can tell you that my clients that eliminate corn from their diet feel relief from many of their emotional and gastrointestinal symptoms. And if you doubt the evidence against all corn, high fructose corn syrup alone is one of the most damaging ingredients in our grocery stores. I have come to believe very passionately in these three things regarding corn:

1. High fructose corn syrup has to be avoided at all cost.

2. Genetically modified corn will continue to prove to be very damaging to our health.

3. Corn oil should never be your first choice when cooking.

RULE #9: AVOID HIGH FRUCTOSE CORN SYRUP AND GENETICALLY MODIFIED CORN

What you can do right now:

1. Divide your pantry. Divide your pantry into foods containing corn and corn byproducts and those food products that are free of high fructose corn syrup.

2. Divide your refrigerator. Do the same in your refrigerator.

3. Eliminate high fructose corn syrup. High fructose corn syrup is one of the most damaging ingredients in our food supply, and you should pay close attention to eliminating foods that contain it.

4. Use and replace. Every time you finish with a product containing genetically modified corn replace it with non-GMO verified corn or replace it with food free of corn altogether. The Non-GMO Project is a non-profit organization that is labeling packaged food.

5. Corn is grain, not a vegetable. When I interview clients on their diets, I repeatedly hear that corn and potatoes are the only two vegetables they are eating. Corn is not a vegetable.

It is a grain. So, when you are planning the vegetables for your family's dinner, make sure you are not planning corn as the vegetable.

6. Buy organic. GMO corn, as discussed in Chapter Three is destructive to our health. If you are going to eat corn in its whole and natural form, such as corn on the cob, make sure you are buying organic corn that is non–GMO. Corn will continue to reveal itself as a significant problem food in our health, but until the information is more mainstream you must at least consume organic. GMO corn is not ever to be trusted when it comes to your health.

CHAPTER TEN

The great white witches, sugar and sweeteners.

$\mathcal{I}$ OFFERED A SEMINAR once on the dangers of sugar, and nobody came. I had many people call and tell me they really wanted to come; they just did not want to know the truth. I know that this is difficult, probably one of the hardest subjects to face, before you skip this chapter, just take a minute to consider how good you might feel with knowing the truth. Remember that knowledge is power, and eventually in our quest for better health we have to face sugar and artificial sweeteners are not bringing us to new heights of health. This chapter was written not to scare you, but to give you power, and the inspiration you need to take complete charge of your health. You will especially need this chapter if sugar or sweeteners have a hold so great over you that you might not see how much it affects the quality of your life.

So powerfully addictive and so prevalent, we do not even want to discuss the possibility that sugar is really bad for us. We have been ignoring warnings for centuries. As early as 1573, we knew there was a correlation between negative behavior and sugar consumption.[128] In spite of early indicators to the negative side of sugar, our health had no fighting chance over our taste buds. Suddenly it became something we had to have, and then it had to be a staple. We became addicted and the long and tumultuous affair with sugar began. Addictive, sweet, and completely problematic to our health, sugar has pushed its way into our lives in extremely massive quantities. It is in just about everything boxed or packaged. Even our health food stores encourage us to believe sugar is okay by having "healthier" versions of sugar called cane juice, or evaporated cane juice, or evaporated cane crystals. Sugar is so addictive in fact, that in scientific experiments, rats would choose sugar over real food when given the choice between the two, and in additional studies rats chose the sugar substitute saccharin over even cocaine.[129] The power of sugar and artificial sweeteners is almost too great to handle, and so our consumption increases.

Most Americans are consuming approximately 140-150 pounds of sugar a year, when the body can only safely handle about ten pounds a year. One hundred and forty pounds of sugar roughly converts to approximately twenty three teaspoons a day.[130] For many, we are not aware of how much we actually consume. Even a seemingly healthy breakfast bar could contain as much as 8 teaspoons of sugar.[131] Many of us do not understand exactly how much sugar we are consuming since food labels use measurements in grams. To identify how many teaspoons of sugar is in a single serving of a packaged food, look at the total grams of sugar listed on the label and divide that number by four.[132] Another way to judge whether a food contains too much sugar is to consider the amount of sugar compared to other ingredients. Ingredients are often listed in the order of the amount, so the first three ingredients make up the most significant amount of the total volume of a food product. If any of the first three to four ingredients are a sugar of some kind, you are getting more than your fair share. Much of the packaged food we consume has too much sugar.

Our addiction starts very young. Baby formulas contain sugar, some contain high fructose corn syrup, and even some organic formulas contain evaporated sugarcane.[133] A child's immune system matures between birth and age two. These are fundamental years where you want to allow your child's immune system to be as strong as possible. If he or she is consuming sugar on a daily basis, his or her immune system may not be maturing adequately leaving them vulnerable for skin conditions such as eczema, food allergies and serious conditions such as asthma. Physical symptoms are only a part of the effect on children consuming high amounts of sugar, emotional symptoms such as hyperactivity, aggressiveness, sadness, and even low self-esteem may all be connected to excessive sugar consumption.[134] I see profound changes in my younger clients' health when parents change sugar consumption from a daily occurrence to one that happens on holidays and special occasions. We have come to believe eating sugar is an integral part of childhood without fully considering the consequences to their health, both physical and mental.

In 1998, the principal of Browns Mill Elementary School of Lithonia, Georgia decided to consider sugar's impact on her school's 20% obesity rate, and just over 50% passing rate on state testing. With the support of parents and the PTA, she replaced candy, soft drinks and sugar snacks, like donut breakfasts, with apples and other kinds of wholesome foods. Principal Sanders-Butler now has a school with no obesity and 80% passing scores on state testing.[135] Also the initiative known as Healthy Kids, Smart Kids has been established, and seventeen other schools have since joined to better the health and performance of their children. So many children are not being allowed to live up to their full potential in school because we fail to make the correlation between what they eat and who they are growing up to be.

Like many adults, most of our children today suffer from a massive sugar addiction. Like the rat that does not understand what is good for him, choosing sugar over food, a child will want what is sweet over most every other food if given the choice. Every time we allow our children to choose sugar snacks, drinks or food in place of wholesome natural foods, we are enabling their addiction and teaching them to disregard their health like allowing them to drive a car before they are old enough to have a license teaches them to disregard safe boundaries and the law. When our children's diet is about what they like and not about what is good for them, we sacrifice their health in order to please them temporarily. As parents we are responsible for growing a healthy and well-adjusted child. Sometimes this means making and standing firm in some hard choices about what we can and cannot eat on a daily basis.

If we struggle with our own addiction, we may not possibly have the strength to deal with the addiction of our children. Until we take charge of our own addiction, we cannot expect to fully take charge of our health or the health of our children. Sugar is linked to more and more health issues every day. Obesity, glucose and insulin response and more recently hyperactivity are a few. Sugar suppresses the immune system, contributes to high levels of trigylcerides and high cholesterol, and is linked to cancers such as ovarian, pancreas and bladder. Sugar is also linked to, cataracts, migraines, PMS, inflammatory conditions such as arthritis and more.[136] Depression in this country is a serious matter. The number of people in this country suffering from depression doubled from the late 90's until now.[137] There has also been a 400% increase in the use of antidepressants in this country since the 1980's, and 11% of Americans, age 12 and over, are taking antidepressants. Unfortunately, statistics note that three times more the population suffers from severe depression and do not even take antidepressants.[138] Sugar consumption contributes to depression because it affects the body's ability to regulate dopamine, serotonin and norepinephrine.[139] Just think our depression epidemic may well be linked to our sugar and artificial sweetener addiction. Giving up sugar can be extremely difficult, but think about what our lives would be like if we gave up sugar and artificial sweeteners on a daily basis. Think about what our entire country would be like if we gave up sugar and artificial sweeteners on a daily basis.

Sugar replacements are not helping us either.

Many people reach for "diet" drinks, and "sugar free" snacks thinking they are making a better choice for their health, but studies reveal artificial sweeteners interfere with our body's appetite control centers, and may even increase hunger.[140] As a result, artificial sweeteners are linked to weight gain. You could say more and more processed food actually stimulates your inability to lose weight. Out of 6,000 new food products to hit store shelves between 1999 and 2004, over 3,600 of these products contained at least one artificial sweetener.[141] That is a lot of artificial sweeteners. Over 15% of us are eating artificial sweeteners on a regular basis.[142] Weight gain and appetite control are a drop in the bucket compared to the questionable safety of these sweeteners.

Aspartame is an artificial sweetener that was given FDA approval in 1974. At that time, scientist Dr. Olney tried to stop the marketing of aspartame in food products, stating he found a correlation between brain tumors and aspartame in rats. He also stated the combination of aspartame and monosodium glutamate could be linked to brain damage in children. This led to an investigation which led a special task force. The task force found more issues and asked for a Senate hearing. In 1977, a grand jury investigation was required. Eventually the charges were dropped because the whole ordeal was just too messy and they could not make heads or tails of any of it. You would think if it was such a mess that they should have been asked to repeat some of the studies. But even though original studies were suspected of fraud and potential illegal activities none of the studies were repeated.[143]

Today aspartame is in over 100 foods. Are we sure the scientific data regarding its safety is accurate? We should never trust such a scandalous substance, no matter what the outcome when there is a possibility that greed and profits motivated approval of this potentially toxic substance. Research the topic yourself, and you will find studies on both sides, one side stating there is still a link to cancer and aspartame, the other side refuting the potential risk to humans. At the end of the day, you can decide for yourself. Aspartame is a profitable substance, exceeding the hundreds of millions in profits yearly.[144]

Sugar and sweeteners are both very problematic. The artificial one is certainly more of a problem than the natural one. But the natural is so excessively consumed that there is a real problem there as well. The truth is you have to begin, slowly if necessary, to bring sugar consumption into moderation. You have to decide your health and your emotional well-being means more to you than the snack or the dessert. It is not easy, in fact the greater the addiction the harder it will be. But there are many good plans and supplements to help you with your addiction. Below are some strategies to help you take action. You will feel better, and each day you feel better and more in control is one more day of success.

RULE #10: AVOID ARTIFICIAL SWEETENERS AND REDUCE SUGAR CONSUMPTION.

What you can do right now:

1. Beware of government approval. When there is too much controversy over whether studies were manipulated for profits, and the risk could be very great to your health, don't consume that particular food. It's that simple. Trust your health to what you know about the laws of nature first.

2. Avoid aspartame, also known as Nutrasweet. It is one of the most controversial artificial sweeteners, and this alone should make you avoid it. Chewing gum is one of the worst. You can also find it in yogurts, sodas and sports drinks. Don't do it, don't let your children do it.

3. The first three ingredients matter most. Avoid sugar in any form when it shows up in the first three ingredients. If sugar, or any variety of sugar, is listed in the first three ingredients, it means that most of what you are eating is sugar. Many times

you can choose a different brand or variety of the food product that doesn't use as much sugar in any form.

4. Natural first. Artificial sweeteners are not a healthier choice. Be careful of labels that say "sugar free." Most likely this means a chemical additive was used. The word "unsweetened" is more likely to have no sugar or artificial sweeteners. To be sure read your ingredients, not just your label.

5. Holidays and parties only. If you limit your sugar consumption to moderate consumption at holidays and special occasions only, you would more than fill your quota of what the body is capable of handling in the way of sugar. Daily consumption carries too great a consequence. Yes, it is effortful, but you and your children are worth the effort.

6. Make your own. Make a commitment that you further limit your sugar consumption down to homemade. If the only way you could eat a cookie was if you made it completely from scratch, how often would you eat them? When making your own, you can also use less sugar than the recipe calls for, or replace the amount of sugar called for in the recipe with ½ that amount of raw honey.

7. By any other name. We derive sweet from a variety of sources, and they all lead to no good. Know their names. Sugar is called by the following: sugar, cane juice, dehydrated cane juice, invert sugar, raw sugar, brown sugar, evaporated cane crystals, molasses, turbinado sugar, raw sugar, and beet sugar. Other kinds of sweeteners, both natural and artificial, include: brown rice syrup, corn syrup, high fructose corn syrup, corn sweetener, corn sugar, dextrin, dextrose, fructose, glucose, maltodextrin, malt syrup, mannitol, rice syrup, saccharose, sorbitol, sorghum, sucrose, splenda, xylose, aspartame, equal, nutrasweet and saccharin.

8. Examine your reasons. Many times sugar is consumed for an emotional reason. If you can ask yourself why you believe you

need the sugar snack or dessert, you have taken the first step. The next step is to ask yourself if there is anything else you can do instead of eating the sugar to help you feel differently. Finding an alternative food or activity can go a long way to distract you. Foods such as a handful of raw almonds, which can give you a protein boost, can help you physically feel better in the moment.

9. One day at a time. The first week of eliminating sugar can be the hardest. In fact, the more of a hold these ingredients have on your body the harder it may be. So take one day at a time. Taking control over something which has control over you, just for one day is one day you have achieved a significant success. Then you can do the next day. And then the next. As the days become weeks and weeks become months, the significance of your success will multiply, and you may be blown away by the improvements your health receives.

CHAPTER ELEVEN

What's in your fat?

$\mathcal{F}$AT IS SUCH a difficult topic. It seems that there have been so many changes in the past several decades over what is good for you and what isn't, how much you should have and how much you should avoid. Before I became a nutritionist, I watched my father obsess about fat free while trying to lose weight. I would cringe at the dedication he had to cutting all fat out of his diet because he believed it was better for him. At the same time, I watched his health suffer from a lack of key nutrients like Vitamin K, which turn out to be fat soluble. Without adequate and healthy fats, Vitamins A, D, E and K are floating around your body without a home. Fat soluble vitamins are dissolved in fat and then stored in fat. We have to have fat, the question is what kind of fat is best and how do we make sure we are getting the highest quality. This chapter will help you have a greater understanding of fats and how to incorporate healthy fats into your meals.

There are three kinds of fat in nature. They are the monounsaturated, polyunsaturated and saturated fats. Monounsaturated and polyunsaturated fats are liquid at room temperature. These are your vegetable oils. Saturated fats are solid at room temperature and are mostly your animal fats (lard, butter, beef and pork fat, etc.) and the plant fats called coconut oil and palm oil. Everyone has heard at least once in their life that high levels of saturated fat are harmful to your health, increasing risk of heart disease. Study after study had linked saturated fat with elevated cholesterol. Then other studies started showing some unusual findings. The first revealed a particular saturated fat, stearic acid, may actually help lower cholesterol instead of raising it.[145] Then more information on polyunsaturated fat starting showing up, and suddenly common vegetable oils may be even more harmful than the saturated fats they had replaced.[146] It really doesn't get any more confusing than that.

It all started when butter, a well-known saturated fat, was given a bad rap, and food manufacturer's came up with a solution called margarine. Most margarine on the shelf today is called spreads, but margarines and spreads are basically the same food. The most harmful of the margarines and spreads are the ones containing hydrogenated or partially hydrogenated oils also known as transfat. Hydrogenation is the manufacturing process of adding hydrogen to the oil in order to keep the oil from spoiling. Transfat is directly linked to the 30,000 or more deaths a year that occur from heart disease and elevated cholesterol.[147] According to the Mayo Clinic, hydrogenated or partially hydrogenated oils are the worst kind of fat because they raise our bad cholesterol and lower our healthy cholesterol.[148] Hydrogenated oils are not just found in certain margarines, they are contained in a variety of processed foods such as chips, cookies, cakes, crackers and peanut butters.

Hydrogen is not the only culprit in the manufacturing of oils. Many polyunsaturated fats like vegetable oils are refined with chemical solvents. These chemical solvents are used to extract the oil from the originating food source and turn a seed or grain into oil. For example, sunflower seeds are turned into sunflower oil. This chemical heating process can put the oil through temperatures as high as 450 degrees, killing off vital nutrients and increasing the chances of these oils becoming transfatty when cooked at home. Even worse, when cooked and reused, usually in restaurants, toxic substances can form in the oil.[149] If your oil does not actually say "cold-pressed," "unrefined" or "extra virgin," then chances are very high that a chemical solvent was used to process the seed or grain into oil.

Many oils are misleading because they "sound" healthier. Vegetable oil containing the word vegetable sounds healthier than lard. But pure lard rendered from animal fat, not the partially hydrogenated oil that is often labeled as lard, contains higher levels of the best fat— monounsaturated fat. Our so called vegetable oils such as canola oil, safflower oil, sunflower oil, soybean oil are all polyunsaturated fats. Polyunsaturated fats are a combination of Omega 3 and 6, but the majority of polyunsaturated fats we consume in this country are heavy with Omega 6 fatty acids. Since our Omega 3 fatty acid consumption is supposed to exceed our Omega 6 consumption for optimal brain, heart and digestive health, the over consumption of vegetable oils rich in Omega 6 is a problem for our health. Polyunsaturated oils have now been linked to chronic inflammation and are also a contributing factor in an Omega 3 deficiency, which most Americans have. Omega 3 deficiencies have been linked to increased risk of inflammation, heart attacks, stroke, asthma, arthritis, headaches, menstrual cramps and osteoporosis.[150]

Since polyunsaturated fat is not the best, and saturated fat is still a problem in excess, the ideal choice is monounsaturated fat. Monounsaturated fat is definitely one of the good guys and can be found in olive oil, walnuts, and avocado. Most monounsaturated fats are rich in Omega 3, which is not only important for blood and heart health, but for the brain as well. Monounsaturated fat helps lower cholesterol and helps prevent heart disease.[151] Sounds pretty good so far. Monounsaturated fats also may help glucose metabolism in individuals at risk for diabetes.[152] We need to eat more monounsaturated fats to help reduce our risk for cholesterol and heart disease and raise our Omega 3 levels. Since most Americans consume far too many processed foods containing polyunsaturated Omega 6, we are in desperate need of more Omega 3. One way to get more monounsaturated fat rich in Omega 3 is to consume more extra virgin olive oil.

Olive oil is one of the most popular monounsaturated fats. Olive oil, due to its monounsaturated fat content and its antioxidant content is also linked to cancer prevention, especially breast and stomach cancer.[153] Mediterranean and other cultures that consume extra virgin olive oil as part of a regular diet often report better heart health. There is no secret to the benefit of olive oil as one of the better choices among oils, but you have to be careful on the quality you purchase. Cold pressed or extra virgin olive oil purchased in dark colored, glass jars is the optimal choice because the oil has not been heated, is not rancid upon purchase and is protected from ultraviolet heat by the colored glass.

Cooking is important as well. The majority of benefits in olive oil will remain constant, if the oil is not heated too high. When we cook with olive oil at high temperatures, we damage the oil because olive oil cannot withstand high heat. This means you can lightly sauté, cooking on a low to medium heat, but you should *not* roast vegetables covered in olive oil at 425 degrees. Cooking on high heat should be avoided as much as possible, but if high heat cooking is required consider alternatives to olive oil. Other healthy fats for cooking include organic pasture fed or grass fed butter if you are consuming cow dairy in moderation, old fashioned (preferably homemade) lard (in moderation), animal fats (when eaten with the muscle such as a steak with marbling—again in moderation), and unrefined coconut oil.

Coconut oil is a great fat for high heat cooking or baking, especially if you are avoiding dairy. Coconut oil has a wonderful way of stimulating metabolism. Lauric acid in coconut oil helps the body balance weight, which means you can assist your body in achieving a more balanced weight either for weight loss or for weight gain.

Coconut oil also contains medium chain triglycerides that increase metabolic energy, which may improve fat oxidation. The combination of the lauric acid and medium chain triglycerides burns the fat you have and replaces that fat with a healthier fat. Therefore you still have to consume coconut oil in moderation because you can lose or gain weight from coconut oil. If you need to gain weight, coconut oil may be beneficial due to its high caloric content and high amounts of saturated fat. One tablespoon of coconut oil contains over 100 calories, with about 12 grams of saturated fat and no cholesterol. The only oil which can be eaten more frequently than coconut oil is olive oil.

Fat is an important part of our diet, responsible for the absorption of fat-soluble vitamins such as Vitamin A, D, E and K. They help insulate organs in the body, and against cold weather. But fat consumption is often abused, and until we are careful in our fat consumption, we run the risk of many chronic and degenerative conditions including inflammation. Inflammation is symptomatic of numerous health related conditions such as arthritis, acne, asthma, autoimmune disease, celiac, and inflammatory bowel disease to name a few. As inflammatory disease rises to epidemic proportions in this country and behavioral disorders affect more and more children each year, we have to take into consideration our fats. If you or someone you love suffers from inflammation, it could very well be related to the kind of fats being eaten. The call of nature again asks us to return to a pure and simpler way of eating where our Omega 3 fats far exceed our polyunsaturated, Omega 6, chemically solvent oils.

RULE #11: CHOOSE GOOD FATS OVER BAD FATS, AND NEVER GO FAT FREE.

What you can do right now:

1. Avoid transfat at all cost. Remember transfat will be called hydrogenated or partially hydrogenated oils on the label. These are the worst of the worst, and you will find transfat most often

in margarine or spreads, soups like Ramen noodles, cake mixes, pancake mixes, frozen food especially pies, cakes and frozen dinners, and fast food. Read your labels very carefully.

2. Seek the virgin. Buy only extra virgin olive oil, this way you can be sure it is cold pressed and nutrients are not lost through a chemical or heat process.

3. Keep it in glass. Buy extra virgin olive oil stored in a colored glass jar. Even the penetration of UV light can begin to break down the oil. Of course, high heat breaks down the oil the worst, so remember to avoid using olive oil on high heat.

4. Make your own. Make salad dressing from scratch with olive oil, and avoid using salad dressing containing inflammatory polyunsaturated vegetable oils such as corn oil, canola oil, safflower oil and soybean oil. Remember most corn oil, canola oil and soybean oil is genetically modified as well.

5. In a rush? If homemade salad dressing does not fit your schedule in the moment, try drizzling extra virgin olive oil or cold pressed flax oil over your salad, and squeeze some fresh lemon juice over the top or add a touch of pink Himalayan sea salt. This will give you a lot of flavor without the trouble of making salad dressing from scratch.

6. Limit high heat cooking. High heat cooking destroys vital nutrients anyway, but when cooking with high heat, consider using pure lard (rendered animal fat, not hydrogenated), organic pasture fed butter or ghee (clarified butter found in many Indian recipes) or unrefined coconut oil.

7. Steam and drizzle. Steaming vegetables in water or lightly sautéing the vegetables in water without overcooking keeps you from worrying about overheating oil. When finished steaming, drizzle the olive oil over the top of the vegetables and sprinkle with sea salt. This way you get all the benefits of the uncooked oil and the entire flavor.

8. Bake at the right temp. Bake with olive oil only if you reduce your baking temperature to 300 degrees, and cook longer to compensate for reducing your heat. Or bake with melted coconut oil or organic pasture butter if you are going to keep the temperature above 300 degrees.

9. Finish right. Have a less expensive extra virgin olive oil for cooking, and use an elegant, more expensive extra virgin olive oil for drizzling over raw or already cooked food. Called finishing oil in some parts of the world, these oils range in texture and taste. When choosing finishing oil look for extra virgin olive oil, imported from Italy, Spain or Greece that has a flavor you like. I found that many of these oils do not have a heavy olive taste that can overpower a meal; instead, they have a light and sometimes fruity taste.

10. Love the coconut fat. Sweeter than most oils, it makes a great choice for baking since it will withstand higher temperatures and adds a sweetness to your dish. Remember that coconut oil will help balance weight for weight gain or weight loss whichever your body needs of this fat you consume.

11. What about flax? Flax seed oil is a great source of Omega 3, and is perfect for salads or in smoothies, but it should never be used for cooking since it can break down in the slightest heat. Flax seed (whole or ground), however, can be used in baking and gives a great crunch to salads, breads or muffins.

PART IV

Let's get real about fruit, veggies, and water.

"Our bodies are our gardens-our wills are our gardeners."
—William Shakespeare

CHAPTER TWELVE

Eat your fruits and veggies.

You REALLY CANNOT achieve optimal health without eating fruits and vegetables, especially vegetables. Hopefully this chapter will inspire you with greater understanding and desire for nature's gifts, fruits and vegetables. Let's begin with vegetables. I've talked a lot about meats, grains, dairy and the dangers of eating those foods, but to the best of my knowledge, no one ever died from eating too many vegetables. There is absolutely no way to be healthy without eating vegetables. Vegetables are the real reason we achieve optimal health through eating—whether we eat meat, don't eat meat, eat dairy or don't eat dairy, eat grains or not. Eating fruits and vegetables have actually been associated with reducing our risk of dying.[154] Without a healthy amount of vegetables on a daily basis, we are asking for disaster. Without eating enough vegetables we are just waiting for the gauntlet of illness and disease to strike. We can change our diet any number of times, but in the end we will feel only as good as the number of vegetables we eat on a daily basis.

What is a vegetable? It is not French fries or potato chips. It is not corn chips or corn. Vegetables are grown out of the ground, whereas most fruit is grown on trees. Yes, potatoes and corn are grown out of the ground, but higher carbohydrate levels in both makes them a starch, and places them in nutritional categories with grains. Vegetables are rich in color such as eggplant, kale, spinach, sweet potato, carrots, and zucchini. Vegetables are healing and cleansing. Vegetables are nature's gift to our health. Vegetables are purifying and nurturing all at the same time. Vegetables contain vitamins, minerals, carbohydrates, essential fatty acids in trace amounts, and yes, even protein. We should pay homage to the almighty vegetable every day—and eat them every day.

The best form of vegetables is raw, or slightly cooked, but never overcooked or burnt. Raw is important for enzyme consumption, but slightly cooked by steaming can increase availability of certain nutrients such as antioxidants. In fact, lightly steaming broccoli can improve not only antioxidants, but also cancer fighting properties.[155] Overcooking is a real problem in most foods and can rob the vegetable of vital nutrients. If you have to eat them, you might as well get the full benefit—otherwise you might have to eat twice as much.

Other ways to get optimal nutrition from your veggies include lightly cooking them in extra virgin olive oil or unrefined coconut oil or lightly steaming them in water. If you lightly steam or sauté vegetables in water, it is important to save the water which contains trace nutrients, and should not be thrown away. A great way to save the liquid is to fill ice trays, freeze in the freezer, and add to soups or casseroles when needing stock. More than anything, do not overcook your vegetables and destroy vital nutrients.

Let's take a look at the nutritional benefits of some specific vegetables. Asparagus is low in calories, but high in protein. Asparagus contains an antioxidant with a history of helping inflammation such as arthritis.[156] Asparagus has also been associated with reducing congestion in the lungs, and improving fertility.[157] Asparagus contains Vitamin A, C and K, potassium, folic acid, riboflavin, thiamin, and B6.

Beets, both the leaves (beet greens) and the beet itself, have a great deal to offer us nutritionally. Beets are traditionally known to improve the health of the liver because it helps the body make glutathione and white blood cells. As a result, beets have now been associated with the fight against colon cancer and stomach cancer.[158]

Another powerful vegetable in the fight against cancer is broccoli. Broccoli is one of the most powerful vegetables nature has ever given us. Even broccoli sprouts pack a lot of nutrients, although some of us would argue that broccoli sprouts are more of an acquired taste. Broccoli contains Vitamin A, C, E, and K, folic acid, B6, potassium, and magnesium. In fact, broccoli contains more Vitamin C than citrus.[159] Broccoli also contains chemicals that help the body fight toxins. One of these chemicals, known as indol-3-carbinol, has been shown to fight breast and prostate cancer cells in early studies.[160]

Cabbage is another superhero in the vegetable kingdom. Cabbage is rich in Vitamin C, E, potassium, calcium, magnesium, manganese, folic acid, B6 and biotin, and Vitamin U, which has been associated with relieving stomach ulcer symptoms.[161] The American Cancer Society also recommends eating plenty of cruciferous vegetables in the fight against cancer such as broccoli, brussel sprouts, and cabbage.[162] Cabbage should be eaten not only steamed, sautéed or raw—but also as fermented sauerkraut. Sauerkraut provides the body with beneficial bacteria and is cleansing to the digestive system.

Most of us know that carrots help with vision due to the high amount of beta carotene contained in this wonderful vegetable, but how many of us understand this powerful vegetable fights against cancer and heart disease as well? In fact, one serving of carrots daily may reduce your risk of heart attack by as much as 60%.[163] And the goodness of beta carotene has been associated with a decrease in the following cancers: bladder, cervical, postmenopausal breast, prostate, and colon.[164] Carrots can also increase the milk supply in nursing mothers, and can help build better teeth in children by decreasing overcrowding.[165] Carrots help eliminate toxins from the body, helping to not only prevent cancer, but also to decrease toxins causing too much stomach acid, too much inflammation, or too much mucus.[166] Carrots can be eaten raw or cooked; in fact, some nutrients are more available by lightly cooking this great vegetable.

Refreshing and light, the cucumber is another magic vegetable. Cleansing to the body, cucumber contains a digestive enzyme to help break down protein and can even help the body eliminate certain kinds of worms that inhabit the intestinal track.[167] Whenever there is mucus of any kind including acne, sore throat, pink eye, cucumber should be added to your diet. Cucumber is rich in silica, the skin nutrient. Silica is a very important nutrient for the skin and connective tissue.[168] Make sure you eat the skin of the cucumber since the skin contains an abundance of minerals including silica, potassium, magnesium and molybdenum.[169]

Underrated and not eaten nearly enough, kale is one of the most important vegetables in the entire family of dark leafy greens. Kale is rich in iron, vitamins and minerals. Kale is also abundant in useable calcium, which makes it a preferred source of calcium for the human body over cow's milk. The power of kale and other dark leafy greens also contain a high concentration of chlorophyll. Chlorophyll could actually be called the essence of life and is a truly important nutrient in the fight against cancer.

Onions add such a wonderful and unique flavor to food, that it is easy to forget the importance of this vegetable. Onion is in the garlic family, and possesses some of the same healing characteristics as garlic such as reducing mucus in the body and helping the immune system. Onions have been linked with lowering blood sugar levels, lowering cholesterol, lowering blood pressure and symptoms associated with asthma.[170]

Spinach is really a super food. Rich in iron and chlorophyll this great food has tremendous ability to purify the blood.[171] Low in calories, but with a nutrient punch, spinach is rich in many B vitamins, magnesium and manganese, Vitamin C, K, and A. The Vitamin A content of spinach along with its lutein content makes this a great food to help with eyesight. There are at least thirteen anticancer and antioxidant components to spinach, making this a go to food for everyone.[172]

Squash, especially winter squash, is not only high in carotenes, which are linked in the fight against cancer, but they also help prevent type 2 diabetes.[173] Squash is rich in many B Vitamins such as folic acid, pantothenic acid, and is a good source of potassium and Vitamin C.[174]

One of the sweeter vegetables is sweet potato, and even though it is considered sweet, it is linked with stabilizing blood sugar levels.[175] Sweet potatoes have tremendous antioxidant properties and contain a plethora of vitamins including Vitamin C, Vitamin B6, fiber, biotin, copper and manganese.[176] They can also help remove toxins in the body when eaten in moderation.[177]

There are many more vegetables abundant in nutrient and health benefits. In spite of the benefits associated with eating vegetables, most Americans do not eat close to what is recommended.[178] When considering nutrition as prevention to illness and disease, vegetables are some of the highest ranking preventative foods. Fruit is important too, but the most important thing to remember about fruit is that it is not a replacement for vegetables.

Eating fruit does not mean a cereal bar with fruit filling, or apple pie, or a pop tart with fruit inside. Fruit is what grows on the tree, and should go from the tree to your hand to your mouth. It is that simple. Fruit is nature's candy. Fruit is cleansing and healing. It is purifying to the body. Fruit contains a wide variety of antioxidants, Vitamin C, bioflavonoids, carotenes and phytochemicals. Fruit has an amazing resume. And it does not stop there. Fruits have been found to protect against cancers, heart disease, cardiac arrest and strokes.[179]

Fruit should be consumed raw and seasonal. Fruit in transport can lose vital nutrients as it ages during its commute from one place to another, such as overseas to your store. So buying local means you improve your chance of eating a fruit with a higher nutrient content.

Buying fruits in season also improves your chances of buying at a better price. Items in season are usually more plentiful and have to be moved off the shelf at a faster rate.

Fruit should also be consumed less frequently than you eat vegetables. Since fruit is sweeter than a vegetable, it is often easier to consume more fruit, and walk away believing we have eaten healthily. Overconsumption of fruit, especially high sugar fruits such as banana and mangoes, can potentially over feed yeast in the body. Fruit sugar is ultimately fructose, and fructose needs to be eaten sparingly.[180] Certainly consuming fructose such as high fructose corn syrup and sucrose table sugar are far more damaging to the body over fruit, but the rule of thumb is to eat twice the amount of vegetables than we eat fruit on a daily basis.

Ideally fruit should be eaten first thing in the morning when the body's digestive system has just completed a cycle of rest and recovery during sleep. And then again, fruit should be eaten in the late afternoon. Fruit is very simple for the body to digest, and because of this simplicity the body will gravitate toward digesting fruit before other foods. This can cause other foods to sit and ferment before key nutrients are absorbed by the body.[181] Ideally, eating fruit first thing in the morning and then later in the day, away from heavier meals such as lunch and dinner, can improve the body's ability to handle fruit sugars.

What we eat in combination with fruit is very important. Fruit when combined with polyunsaturated oils, processed foods made from flour, or certain proteins can also potentially create toxins in the body.[182] What does that mean? Well, for one thing the fruit cereal bar is not as healthy as you believe, and the deep fried apple pie at a fast food restaurant is very unhealthy. And eating a hot dog or hamburger on a bun and following it with watermelon is a real problem for the body. So, avoid processed snacks containing fruit, and avoid fruit at the same meal with processed meats.

There is one last major consideration in fruit consumption. Fruit juices sold in boxes and bottles (glass or plastic) are not good for us. Just because we think these are natural does not mean they should be consumed. Fruit juice can contain high amounts of natural sugars even if the container says "not from concentrate" "low sugar" or "fortified." Pasteurization in fruit juice also destroys valuable enzymes necessary to break down fruit sugars—even if those sugars are naturally occurring fruit sugars. Water is the true drink of nature, and is addressed later in Chapter Fifteen.

Fruit has incredible health benefits. Fruit consumption has been linked to the reduction of certain cancers.[183] There are so many different and wonderful fruits, but the apple is the single most important fruit we should eat. The saying, "An apple a day keeps the doctor away" actually was a clever way to remember the complete and magnificent benefits of this fruit. Apple alone (organic with the skin on) contains calcium phosphate, iron phosphate, potassium phosphate, magnesium phosphate, and sodium phosphate making it the only food on the planet that contains all these nutrients. An apple is the perfect food for making energy in the body. An apple also contains quercetin, an ingredient that helps reduce mucus buildup in the body. Apples have been proven, in not just one study but over 85 different studies, to reduce risk of cancer, heart disease, asthma and diabetes.[184] In addition to apples, fruits such as blueberries, peaches, strawberries, and pears are just a few of nature's candy offering antioxidants and bioflavonoids to help us stay fit and healthy.

Unfortunately, one of the concerns we need to have with eating fruit is the level of pesticides and herbicides found in the very insides of these wonderful foods. According to the Environmental Working Group (EWG) 2011 report on pesticides and food, apples are ranked number one in the highest number of pesticides.[185] Remember the benefits of fruits are tremendous. With the knowledge of how to grocery shop safely, as discussed in Chapter Two, and how to eat fruit and combine it with other foods appropriately, you can enjoy the sweetest of nature's foods without worry.

Rule #12: Eat fruits and veggies daily, but eat twice as many vegetables as you do fruit.

What you can do right now:

1. Try raw spinach. Spinach is one of the most comprehensive nutrients on the planet. There are plenty of interesting and exciting ways to eat spinach. Try raw spinach combined with sliced strawberries—with or without dressing. Or try raw spinach with sliced pears, raw pecans and goat feta. Another time try adding sliced red onion and sautéed mushrooms. The possibilities are endless and so is the improvement to your health.

2. Eat broccoli. Preliminary research studies indicate eating two pounds of broccoli a week can reduce your risk of cancer by as much as fifty percent.[186] Two pounds is a lot, but you can do tremendous benefit by committing to eating broccoli at least once a week and increasing your consumption from there. Broccoli can be steamed and served as a side, or chopped raw added to salads.

3. Remember your quota. You must eat a minimum of four servings of vegetables a day. A serving is a ½ cup. Four servings is two cups and very doable.

4. Nature's Bounty. Here are some great tidbits for adding variety as you strive to meet your quota. Asparagus is best in the spring, and can be eaten raw, or sautéed in olive oil with a touch of sea salt. Beets are most commonly found in a soup called borscht, but have a lot more versatility. Great ideas for eating beets include shredding raw beets into salads, or roasting beets and then drizzling with olive oil and sprinkle with goat feta cheese. Try these different ways to eat cabbage: 1.) Cook in a crock-pot with onion, potatoes and bison sausage, 2.) Make into raw coleslaw made with apple cider vinegar and olive oil,

3.) Shredded raw into fish tacos in place of lettuce, or 4.) Add sauerkraut alone or added to homemade soups. Sweet potato or winter squash can be baked then drizzled with olive oil and sprinkled with sea salt. Or try grating raw butternut squash in a salad for something new. The opportunities for vegetables in your diet are endless.

5. Eat an apple a day. Any kind will do. Each variety has a slightly different texture and flavor, so you can pick tart, sweet, mild, or crunchy. First thing in the morning on an empty stomach is the ideal time to eat an apple; but any time you slice it, you toast your health every time you eat one organic apple with the skin on.

6. Raw for snacking. When reaching for an afternoon snack, a piece of raw fruit will benefit your health, and your energy levels. Fresh fruit carries more nutrients than a fruit "snack." Fruit snacks such as fruit bars, fruit strips and gummies have fewer nutrients, and may be more complicated to digest if containing refined carbohydrates such as white flour and vegetable oils.

7. Watch the invisibles. Since we are more inclined to eat a piece of fruit directly out of the refrigerator, it is very important to wash fruit before you eat it. Washing will help remove any invisible organisms lingering on the outside of the fruit. What you do not see, can hurt you.

8. Partner correctly. Make sure when eating fruit, you try to avoid the combination of fruit and artificial ingredients, fruit and white flour or fruit and refined sugar. Try a piece of raw fruit combined with a handful of raw nuts. Apple with almonds and pears with pecans are some lovely combinations.

9. Sweet and the meat. Watch and avoid the combination of processed meats and fruit. This means you should avoid fruit with meats such as bacon, ham, cold cuts, and hot dogs.

10. Shred and hide, if needed. If you or your child is a picky eater,

no one should be indulged and given the opportunity to avoid vital nutrients. In this situation, it is very important to find strategies to help introduce vegetables into the diet until they are a regular part of eating. One such strategy is shredding vegetables such as zucchini, carrots, onion and spinach and adding them to meatloafs, muffins, pancakes and quiches. Over time your taste buds will enjoy the taste of vegetables more.

11. Dark smoothies. Another great place to add more vegetables is to make smoothies. When you make a smoothie with strawberries, blackberries or blueberries they are dark enough to hide dark leafy greens and the sweetness of the smoothie helps offset the taste of the greens. Spinach and kale are easy additions to a fruit smoothie with not a lot of bitter aftertaste.

12. Watch the juice. Bottled and boxed fruit juice should be avoided. Bottled and boxed fruit juice often breeds bacteria and has tested positive for some of the same contaminants in tap water. Homemade juices are a much safer choice.

13. Healing your taste buds. Our taste buds can literally be destroyed by the sugars and sodium in processed foods causing us to further crave saltier and sweeter foods. This perpetuates a cycle where we avoid whole and healthy foods because they are not salty or sweet enough. If whole fruits and vegetables are something you do not like the taste of you very likely have deadened taste buds. Give your taste buds the chance to heal if they are damaged. And the only way to do this is to stop the cycle of eating salty and sugary foods. Once you are eating less processed foods, your taste buds will come back to life again and enjoy the sweetness of fruits and vegetables without the sugar and salt.

14. Add pink. Pink Himalayan sea salt added to steamed or sautéed vegetables will add extra minerals and enhance the flavor of food.

CHAPTER THIRTEEN

Acid is for batteries

I LOVE THE SOPHISTICATION of the human body. We have come so far in understanding the body's complexities that we now know our bodies are far more intricate than any machine. Yet, there is still so much more we do not know. And when it comes to nutrition there are so many different positions. I have been studying food, nutrition and natural living for over fifteen years now, and I am still in awe of the constantly changing information about what is good for us to eat. Certain diets work for some people and not for others. There are those that do better on vegetarian lifestyle than others. Others are healthier as meat eaters. I believe the reason why different individuals achieve different results on certain diets may actually be very simple, but one that is often missed. This chapter is about connecting the dots, and bringing everything about food together under one fundamental rule. Balancing combinations of acidic and alkaline foods in our diets has more influence on our health than the food pyramid method or other methods of structuring our diet.

This acid alkaline balance is really one of the greatest secrets to wellness through nutrition and diet. If the acid alkaline balance was better understood, we could more easily navigate through and around the toxic world we live in and make better choices. When this fundamental truth is ignored, then it does not matter what foods we eat we will eventually put ourselves in great risk of health consequences. Simply put, the amount of alkaline foods we eat helps our bodies deal appropriately with the amount of acidic foods we eat. Consuming more quality alkaline foods over acidic foods can take our health to a greater level. Let's take a look at what that means exactly.

You may remember these terms from a junior high or high school science class. Anything we ingest can be labeled as an acid or an alkaline based on the effect it will have on pH levels, or measurements, in bodily fluids and solids like urine, saliva, blood and stool. When our blood baseline is too acidic the body makes adjustments to make sure our blood remains slightly alkaline. When the body makes these corrections, our urine, saliva and stool may become too acidic. This continual state of acidity in the urine is known as metabolic acidosis. When metabolic acidosis occurs we may be more vulnerable to illness and disease. How does this happen? In simple terms, the food we eat may either lower our metabolic pH making us more acidic, or elevate our metabolic pH making us more alkaline. Again, when pH is lowered we become more acidic, and when pH is elevated we become more alkaline. Through the course of the day our metabolic pH may fluctuate up and down based on what we ingest and our stress levels. This is normal. The damage comes if we repeatedly lower our metabolic pH and then fail to raise it again. This can happen if the basis of our diet is acidic over a long period of time. Eating too much or too many acidic foods will keep our metabolic pH low. Over the long term, what we eat on a day-to-day basis is a huge part of how vulnerable we are to illness and disease.

All foods and other non-food ingredients that we ingest will either raise or lower our pH level. So, we can theoretically categorize what we consume as either an acidic food or an alkaline food. In general, most fruits (except cranberries, dates and figs), most vegetables (except peas), nuts (except peanuts, pecans and walnuts) and seeds will have an alkaline effect on our internal pH. Grains (except oats, quinoa and millet), meats, beans (except lentils), cooking vegetable oils (except olive oil and coconut oil which are alkaline) and certainly all non-food items such as pesticides, pharmaceuticals and chemical additives will have an acidic effect on our internal pH. This alkaline and acidic effect is not dependent on whether a food's own pH is acidic, like lemon, tomato or orange juice. What we are considering is the effect on our internal pH, and a lemon is actually one of the most powerfully alkaline foods.

When you think about the fact that all meats and refined carbohydrates made from grains are on the acidic side most Americans are consuming a highly acidic diet. Over time, this highly acidic diet causes us to become more vulnerable to illness and disease. Vital nutrients such as calcium, magnesium, and potassium are not available in a highly acidic diet. They are supposed to be supplied by alkaline foods in order to neutralize the acidic foods.

If we do not supply the alkalinity through food, such as vegetables and fruits then the body will look for alkalinity elsewhere. It will find it stored in our body, in our bones and joints, and it will take these nutrients to help neutralize acidic food. Literally, our bodies will attempt to save itself from the harmful affects of acidic foods by leeching nutrients right out of our bones, tissues and joints. Remember the body needs to keep the blood pH at a certain place, and if this is not achieved through diet, the body will find these minerals in reserves. Once alkaline minerals are used to neutralize our acidic diet, these nutrients are not kept for good use in the body. Instead, they get dumped in the kidneys and excreted in our urine.[187] This leeching of nutrients from our bones and muscles and tissues, make us more vulnerable to conditions such as osteoporosis.[188] In fact, it has been proven in over 100 studies that the more fruits and vegetables you consume, the greater your bone density.[189]

If you eat a predominantly acidic diet you may experience constipation, mood issues, sleep issues, focus issues, leg cramps, painful joints, stiffness, fatigue, among many more symptoms and not even realize that these symptoms are related to the food you are eating. You're wondering what these issues have to do with an acidic diet. Take constipation. Your body needs extra magnesium to help neutralize acidic foods. Magnesium deficiencies are often related to constipation. Magnesium and calcium deficiencies are often related to mood and behavioral issues due to the calming effect of magnesium and calcium on the body. This is also a great example of why eating is such a powerful aspect to our health. We can actually eat food to raise our metabolic pH, strengthen our bodies, calm and focus ourselves, and help ourselves become more resistant to illness and disease.

The body will strive to correct and balance itself, if our diet is rich with alkaline foods. Our metabolic pH becomes more alkaline, and we can balance the health of the body. There are several ways of improving pH. The first step to improving our pH is through a cleansing diet. Cleansing our body by eating only alkaline foods for seven consecutive days and then maintaining an alkaline dominant diet may be what you need to improve your health. Another way to improve your alkalinity is to make sure the number of alkaline food outnumber the acidic food at each meal. Lastly, make sure that, by the end the day, your total consumption of food is more alkaline.

Ideally your day should consist of 60% alkaline foods and no more than 40% acidic foods.[190] If you are trying to significantly improve your health or reach a particular health goal, then 80% alkaline and 20% acidic is truly needed. The typical American diet is reverse of what is needed. All too often, individuals are eating 10-20% alkaline (if they are somewhat aware) and 80-90% acidic. One of the most profound moments for my clients is when their food diary is scored according to the number of alkaline and acidic foods. Each and every client is amazed when they see how few alkaline foods they are eating through the course of a day. You can try it home. Keep record of your food for three days. Then tally up the alkaline foods and then the acidic foods. Compare the two categories. Examine what your ratio of alkaline to acidic foods. Remember you need to have more alkaline foods over acidic.

Like most of my clients, you will likely be appalled at the amount of alkaline foods you are failing to eat. If you eat hardly any alkaline foods, you will need a place to begin; otherwise, you will give up. Until you are accustomed to eating an alkaline dominant diet, eating more alkaline foods will not be desirable or easy. Taking baby steps will help you transition and improve your chances of making a permanent change. Eating alkaline dominant should be a lasting part of your lifestyle and not a fad.

For beginners it is very simple—make sure each time you have a meal it contains an alkaline food. Then eventually you should work toward a 50/50 split, where for every acidic portion there is an alkaline portion. By doing this you are eating enough alkaline foods at every meal to neutralize the acidic foods that may be on your plate. An example of eating with awareness to the acid alkaline balance is having chicken (acid) with two kinds of vegetables (alkaline), and baked potato (alkaline) instead of chicken (acid) and pasta (acid) and cream sauce (acidic). It really is not as complicated as it seems, it just takes a little understanding and some creativity.

Improving your metabolic pH is much easier once you make some of the initial changes suggested in this book, such as eating quality meat and organic produce. When you add more alkaline foods, you are taking complete charge of your nutritional health and not just reducing the toxic load. It very easy to believe we are eating healthy and instead slip into an acidic state. Hummus and rice crackers on the surface can seem healthy enough, but both are acidic, so a little reorganization of hummus with apple slices or carrot sticks, or a completely alkaline snack of cashews with sliced pear can relieve some the acidic stress affecting the body.

Remember acid foods include meat, almost all grains, most cooking oils, almost all legumes, and dairy, pasta, condiments, peanuts, pesticides and pharmaceuticals. Alkaline foods include vegetables, most fruits, seeds, spices, almonds, cashews, lentils, garlic, apple cider vinegar and herbal teas.[191] At the end of the book is a handy chart to help you follow acid and alkaline food. Understanding acid alkaline balance is not just good eating, it is a fundamental belief that defines a solid foundation to your good health through nutrition. Let's face it. No one ever said someone developed high cholesterol or heart disease or obesity because they ate too many vegetables. We can keep looking for justifications to eat poorly or find some fad diet that says it is okay to have chocolate cake every day; but in doing so we spin ourselves into circles without feeling any better. Here are some fallacies we have come to when we deny the importance of the acid alkaline balance.

1. Myth: Counting calories is the way to lose or gain weight.

    You may lose weight initially but keeping it off may remain a real problem if you never learn how to organize your fruits and vegetables adequately against your meats and grains. Alkaline foods metabolize in the body much faster than acidic foods, and they help our body metabolize the acidic foods better.

2. Myth: Vegan or vegetarian is better.

    If we become vegetarian, and relieve ourselves of toxic animal products we can feel better initially in what is known as a detoxification phase. But, if we replace meat with a lot of grains (acidic) and not enough vegetables (alkaline) our results from a vegetarian lifestyle will be short lived.

3. Myth: Eating meat is better.

    Again, if our diet is mostly protein (acidic) without the fruits, vegetables and healthy fats (alkaline,) our health may suffer greatly. We benefit from meat based on its quality and how well we balance its consumption with vegetables.

    We can argue the merits of eating a variety of diets, but different philosophies truly work, or do not work, based on an individual's intake of whole alkaline foods. A balanced diet, where the majority of foods consumed are whole and alkaline based is the fundamental truth to healthy eating. Without eating enough whole alkaline foods, it does not matter if we eat meat or not, eat dairy or not, eat organic or not, we will be lost nutritionally.

RULE #13: EAT THE ACID ALKALINE BALANCE OF AT LEAST 60/40.

What you can do right now:

1. Begin with one meal at a time. Focus on one meal at a time until you get the hang of it. For some people starting with dinner is best, because you might be more likely to make better choices for the whole family. For others dinner is too stressful a time to be the starting place. At your chosen meal, limit the number of acidic food, ingredients, and condiments at that particular meal down to one or two acidic foods. Fill the remainder of the plate with alkaline foods. Remember, processed foods contain acidic ingredients like white flour and sugar in addition to the base ingredients, and many condiments are acidic. Also remember, most oils are acidic and keeping to healthy fats such as extra virgin olive oil and unrefined coconut oil plays an important part of your diet. Example: You might be currently eating this: pasta (acidic), chicken (acidic), white sauce (acidic) and broccoli (alkaline) in the same meal. Now change it to this: pasta (acidic) tossed with olive oil (alkaline) and sautéed vegetables such as onion, red bell pepper, zucchini and mushroom (alkaline) and chicken breast (sparingly to keep the ratio of vegetables higher in quantity).

2. Rethink other meals. Once you have mastered the first meal, begin to allow this eating philosophy to spill over into other meals. One quick tip for making the transition—any time you eat an acidic food such as meat or grain or dairy, serve a vegetable.

3. Rethink the day. You may find that arranging each meal is too difficult, and just cannot start your day in any other way than with a traditional breakfast. Solution: Make sure your total alkaline foods outnumber your total acidic food by the end of the day. This means if you eat eggs and sausage for breakfast, you can still do fine if you have fruit for a morning snack or a large salad for lunch. You can still achieve the desired amount of alkaline foods by the end of the day if you look toward an end of the day goal.

4. Measure your results: You can see first hand what your pH is through a simple at-home test using pH strips. First morning urine is best for determining overall pH since recent food consumption and daily stress will affect your pH and may not give you a clear picture of your resting pH. Morning urine pH range of anywhere between 6.5-7.0 is ideal and anything lower may indicate an acidic state. A visualization of your own metabolic acidity is a powerful tool. Improving your pH and watching the improvement is highly motivating as well.

5. Accelerate results. You can do three things through the course of the day to help improve pH very rapidly. One, consume lemon water made from fresh lemons (very alkaline) and filtered water. Squeeze one half of a lemon in 8 ounces of filtered water and drink this first thing in the morning on an empty stomach. Two, consume 1 teaspoon of unfiltered apple cider vinegar in 8 ounces of filtered water in the late afternoon for 1-2 weeks at a time to help bring pH back to normal in addition to dietary changes. Three, potassium is a great alkalizing nutrient. Eating food rich in potassium such as avocados, pistachios, bananas, dried apricots and pumpkin seeds will go a long way to help your pH. This also, in addition to dietary changes, helps neutralize the acidity in the body.

CHAPTER FOURTEEN

Red, green and raw.

$\mathcal{E}$ ATING HEALTHY IS a journey and should be taken in manageable steps. As the saying goes, "Rome was not built in a day." You too, should not take on every single change at once. As I share with my clients, eating is not just about food, but a part of the way we live our lives. Plus, if you made all these changes in your house at once, anyone who is living with you may turn against you. Or if you yourself take on too many changes at once, you may give up. We live in a culture where so much is easy and requires so little effort, that if you do not take it one step at a time it may become too much work and you will go back to an easier way. But if you take one step at a time, once you have mastered each step, you will want to take the next step because you will feel so good. This chapter is the next two steps—eating colorful and eating raw. This is easier than you might think, and of course you have to have strategies to help you along the way. Let's begin with color.

Color is a very important strategy in creating healthy meals. A meal based in color can help you achieve greater health and wellness. Eat the rainbow is not a new or novel idea, but for some it may be too broad an idea. Eating the rainbow does not mean we have to eat all the colors of the rainbow at every meal. Purple is a color in very few foods. In simpler terms, you need to eat red, which includes shades of red such as orange, yellow and peach colored foods, and green at main meals. Eating reds and greens means you get food rich in antioxidants, bioflavonoids, vitamins, minerals, and enzymes. Eating red and green also means greater alkaline food at your meal. Eating red and green is absolutely fundamental to your health and will take your meals to the next level. Eating red and green is a small tip that packs a lot of punch.

Here are some of your green foods: Kale, chard, spinach, lettuce, cucumbers, zucchini, asparagus, broccoli, arugula, avocado, green beans and peas. Here is some of your red, orange and yellow food: tomatoes, acorn squash, butternut squash, sweet potato, beets, red bell pepper, apple, strawberries, peaches, and cantaloupe. Making sure you have red and green at main meals will also improve the visual appearance of your meals. You will be pleasantly surprised how much more appreciative your family is with the tasty looking, as well as healthy, meal you have served. After making sure you have the red and green colors working for you at main meals, you will want to understand raw food and how this fits into the big picture.

After you have committed to real food, have changed the quality of your food, have increased your alkaline foods, and incorporated color foods at main meals, you are ready to talk about balancing raw foods with cooked foods. Most people consume far too many cooked or processed (which is essentially cooked) foods and not enough raw foods. Others follow a raw food philosophy that promotes eating a completely raw diet. This type of diet is far too limiting for the average individual and not very practical if you want to participate in the current culture. Also such a diet negates some of the benefits that certain foods gain once they are cooked, so again balance is important.

Ideally, you should have a serving of raw fruit or vegetable at each meal to maintain a good balance between raw and cooked foods in your diet. For the sake of our health, we need a balance of cooked and raw foods. The most important reason to maintain this balance is to ensure good digestion.

The human body relies on three categories of enzymes to help the body run optimally—digestive enzymes (which are made by the body), metabolic enzymes (which help the body run), and food enzymes (which are found only in raw food.) All three of these enzyme groupings are the necessary healthy trio of good digestion. We cannot have optimal health if we only make enzymes in our body and fail to consume food enzymes. If we do not consume enough food enzymes, the body lacks optimal digestion. And if we do not make enough digestive enzymes, we cannot have optimal health.

The digestive process includes a host of enzymes that help break down food. The first of these digestive enzymes are released in our saliva when we chew and grind our food. Chewing is a very important step in our digestive process because our mouth is where we begin to break down food by mixing it with saliva. Saliva is not only for lubricating food. It also contains enzymes, such as amylase, to assist with carbohydrate digestion. Without digestive enzymes generated in our saliva, stomach, small intestine, pancreas and liver, our body would not be able to digest carbohydrates, proteins and fats effectively.[192] A healthy digestive system allows the body to take what it needs and eliminate the waste through urine and feces. When our digestive system does not run optimally, we may have a difficult time eliminating waste, which may stress our colons, our immune system, our liver, our circulatory system and our kidneys.[193]

Stress on our colons can manifest in constipation. Constipation is so common in developed countries that most people believe it to be normal. But common does not make something normal. We are constipated so often because we do not understand what "healthy" means when referring to a healthy colon or a healthy number of bowel movements. Consider this, if digestion includes the process of eating and eliminating, then it would make sense to eliminate after a main meal. If the body detoxifies and filters while we sleep, then it would make sense that the largest bowel movement of the day would be within one to two hours after rising in the morning. One easy to pass, large bowel movement in the morning and at least one to two more bowel movements throughout the day (preferably within an hour of a main meal) is one major indicator that you are experiencing a healthy digestive system and healthy colon. And if you are experiencing less than that, the reality is you are constipated.

Aside from any serious health problems or illness, your constipation may very well be associated with any of the following:

» A lack of real and wholesome food, such as not enough fruits, vegetables and fiber.

» Eating too many refined carbohydrates, especially when combined with proteins or with fruit.

» Too much of an acid base in the body where minerals such magnesium are no longer in abundance.

» Eating too much cooked food.[194]

Cooked food, especially overcooked food, is depleted of important vitamins and minerals during the cooking process that were contained in its original raw form. Cooked food can also cause the body to experience an elevated white blood cell count, especially when we eat too much cooked, processed food.[195] To the contrary, raw food is rich in vitamins, minerals and food enzymes. Raw food enzymes, such as cellulase, help the body break down fiber.[196] We need the fiber to help us stay regular, but we also need the enzymes to help break down the fiber. This makes raw food an essential ingredient in our daily regime.

Food enzymes are a very interesting process in fruits and vegetables, which we often misperceive the beginning work of food enzymes as food going bad. At some point all fruits and vegetables decompose into a state that is no longer acceptable to eat, but the beginning stages of decomposition is food enzymes at work. When we bite or cut into a piece of fruit, such as an apple or a pear, and we see that some spots are brown we need to understand that the enzymes our bodies need are starting to do their job. If we then eat that fruit, we will benefit from those enzymes. As the enzymes become activated, they break the cellular wall within the fruit, and we see the resulting color change. Once we eat the fruit these enzymes mix with digestive enzymes in our saliva and activate our metabolic enzymes. When this amazing trio of enzymes happens we benefit from all the nutrients the raw food contains.

This beautiful symphony of enzymes in food and enzymes within our body create the beautiful music of digestion. A healthy digestive system should be something we strive for because factors, such as poor diet and age, can actually deplete our enzyme efficiency. The combination of a poor diet and the aging process can cause our body to decrease its enzyme production. We cannot stop the aging process, but we can slow the decrease in our enzyme production by paying closer attention to our diet. We can improve our body's enzyme production by eating more raw food. Especially as we age, there are too many health consequences of a diet filled primarily with cooked food. In order to achieve better health, we have to eat more raw food.

Many people have embraced what is a called a raw food diet to achieve this abundance of enzymes and gain greater health. What exactly is a raw food diet? There is a lot of misunderstanding about a raw food diet. It does not mean we only eat salads. A raw food diet means we eat raw food and cook food at a temperature no higher than 115 degrees Fahrenheit to preserve all the vitamins, minerals and enzymes in those foods. For many of us, this is too involved a process to be able to maintain our current lifestyle. But we cannot throw out the facts just because we do not have the time or the understanding. Raw food is an essential part of a healthy diet and needs to be consumed every day, but does not necessarily have to be the only way we eat. We need to be mindful of the how high our cooking temperatures are, limiting our high heat cooking such as boiling, high heat roasting, grilling and broiling. We can also achieve some of the benefits of a raw food diet by cooking lightly, such as steaming or sautéing, and adding a serving of raw food to every meal. Eating raw at every meal means you can still prepare many of the traditional meals you are accustomed to with small adjustments to help you receive tremendous health benefits.

Examples of adding raw to your meal:

1. Oatmeal with raw strawberries, raw sunflower seeds, and raw sliced almonds with raw unfiltered honey. (add a teaspoon of dehydrated seaweed for your "green")

2. Omelet with sliced raw tomato, and raw avocado on the side. Or diced tomato and green onion (or red) sprinkled on top of the omelet after cooked.

3. Romaine lettuce salad with shredded raw carrots, sliced raw tomato and raw cucumber and grilled chicken breast, roasted potatoes and asparagus.

4. Rice pasta with sautéed vegetables such as onion, zucchini, mushroom and red bell pepper, with raw spinach salad of spinach, raw red onion, raw pecans and sliced raw pear.

5. Buffalo or grass fed steak, sautéed broccoli, baked potato with raw chives, diced raw red onion, and sliced tomato salad with raw sliced tomato and fresh raw basil.

RULE #14: EAT RED, GREEN AND RAW AT EVERY MEAL.

What you can do right now:

1. Pick one. Pick a favorite fruit or vegetable and try to combine that favorite with one food you are not crazy about in the opposite color. For example, if you like strawberries but are not crazy about leafy greens, try a salad with spinach leaves and sliced strawberries. A winning combination.

2. Don't allow color dominance. It is easy to choose one color and have that be the dominant color to your meal. Pasta with tomato sauce or steak with potato and broccoli are two examples of one color dominance. You can improve your nutritional value to your meal by looking for the opportunity to add another color to a one color dominant meal. For example, steak with sweet potato, broccoli and side salad with lettuce and tomato is a more colorful and more nutritionally complete meal. The meal of pasta with a zucchini, mushroom and onion tomato sauce with side salad of mixed greens and shredded carrot is more nutritionally complete.

3. Be creative. Adding the color can be a quick add-on to any given meal, it does not need to be a complete side dish or involve a lot of preparation. For example, say you have finished preparing a roast chicken, and you are going to serve it with rice and broccoli. And at the last minute you realize you have no red food, and you do not want to make another side dish. You can very quickly add the color to your plate, with several options:

   a. You can shred raw carrot into the rice along with a green or red onion. By shredding or dicing very small you can add this ingredient at the last minute and keep it raw.

   b. You can slice red bell pepper and serve on the side, or chopped and into the rice.

   c. You can slice raw tomatoes and drizzle with extra virgin olive oil, sprinkled with sea salt and pepper and serve it on the side. Or you can add a touch of lemon juice or balsamic vinegar with the olive oil if you do not want the flavor of the olive oil and salt alone.

    d. A quick tomato salad can also be served with tomatoes alone, or you can throw some fresh or dried basil to give it some kick. You can also slice red onion very thin and combine with the tomatoes.

4. Make a promise. Promise yourself and your health that you will eat a raw food at every meal. When preparing a meal, choose a raw food first, so you don't forget.

5. Prep ahead. Don't forget pre-cut and pre-washed leafy greens make eating a salad easy as one-two-three. Washing and cutting as part of unpacking your groceries makes access to raw vegetables quick and easy.

6. Snacks can be easy. Snacks are a great way to pick up extra servings of raw foods. Raw fruits such as apples, pears, and berries. Or raw nuts, such as almonds, walnuts and pecans. Or carrots sticks, celery sticks or sliced radishes.

7. Last minute add-ons. You can add a raw vegetable at the last minute to any meal. Examples are shredded carrots. These can be added to any soup, salad, rice or vegetable dish. Or green onions or chives that can be diced and added to meats, potatoes or salads.

8. Be a treat to the eyes and the tummy. Color and raw means your plate is a real treat for the eyes and your health.

CHAPTER FIFTEEN

Clean water, please.

WHENEVER I SHARE with a client their symptoms may be related to not enough water, there is a look of confusion on their face. It seems like too simple an answer to ease some of the pain or the stiffness or the constipation or the severe headaches. Yet, this simple gift from nature, of hydrogen and oxygen is so good for our bodies. Water is a powerful and necessary part of our health and is often overlooked. But it must be pure and clean water, because the alternative of contaminated, unclean water can often cause many problems. Drinking pure clean water is actually one of the most significant nutritional decisions you can make for your health for the very reason we are mostly water. The human body is half, or more than half, water. Children are approximately 70% water, and adults between 50% and 60% water. As babies in the womb we are actually 80% water. But just turning on the tap or hydrating ourselves with coffee and juice is turning a blind eye to a fundamental key to our health, so this chapter focuses on both the quality and quantity of our water.

Water is contained in all our bodily fluids from blood to urine to tears. Water is also part of almost every system in the body from digestion to elimination. The average adult will lose approximately two quarts of water per day through sweat and urine. Thus, we have a tremendous need to replenish the water lost from our bodies. When we fail to replenish the water lost throughout the day, we may experience symptoms associated with diabetes, arthritis, back pain, joint pain, chronic fatigue, depression, constipation and headaches to name a few.[197] If we further deplete the body and become dehydrated, we can experience even greater health issues. Some of our rehydration comes to us through the water content of fruits and vegetables. The rest of it comes from the water we drink, and many of us fail to consider the risks involved with drinking ordinary tap water.

For many of us, pure clean water may be more elusive than we think. Many Americans are buying bottled water because it is convenient, easy to buy, and we are convinced it is a healthier choice over tap water. Bottled water is so popular and trendy it leads the sales in bottled beverages. Currently, we are drinking about 30 billion bottles totaling 8.6 billion gallons of water annually,[198] but most bottled water contains higher amounts of bacteria over tap water. In fact, most bottled water does not even meet the safety regulations of tap water, but clever marketing leads us to think bottled water is cleaner.[199] However, bottled water is not, by a long shot, a cleaner healthier version of water. In a documentary called *Tapped* viewers are informed of Nestle® bottled water being sourced from several municipal water sources in the state of Maine, revealing that many of the bottled water we buy is only filtered tap water.[200] And tap water is very concerning.

Currently tap water is regulated by the Environmental Protection Agency (EPA) with the National Primary Drinking Water Standards and voluntary compliance to Secondary Drinking Water Standards added in 1992.[201] The EPA monitors potential contamination of over 80 different toxic substances that can be present in our drinking water at any given time. The US Geological Survey also monitors additional pesticides, bacteria and other toxins that can be present in our drinking water.[202]

But having regulations and following them are two different things. As many as forty two states have been cited with repeated violations of these regulations with contaminants exceeding allowable levels from excessive pesticides to excessive chlorination byproducts.[203] Regulations aside, there are still concerning issues to be discussed. In 2003, in a water report from the Agency for Toxic Substances and Disease Registry the most concerning substances in our drinking water are lead, arsenic, mercury, vinyl chloride and PCB's (polychlorinated biphenyls).[204] Some of these substances need to be understood further.

One concern is our exposure to lead. Lead contamination through drinking water may be affecting as many as 40 million Americans.[205] We are exposed to lead through the lead content of the pipes our drinking water runs through constantly. Lead is leeched from the pipes because water is treated with chemicals that are corrosive.[206] Since 1985, tap water has been known by environmentalists to be a major source of lead. There does not seem to be a direct solution, boiling water will help with some water contaminants, but even boiling the water does not eliminate our exposure to lead. Children seem to be the most vulnerable absorbing as much as 50% of the lead they drink where it will be stored in tissues, circulated in the bloodstream, and is linked to cognitive damage.[207]

The older the city, the older the pipes and this increases our risk to lead exposure. Several states in New England have struggled with lead in its drinking water for some time due to aging pipes. Rhode Island now monitors their water closely after a significant number of children tested positive for three times the amount of allowable lead in their drinking water. Oregon, which has some of the most proactive water regulations regarding lead, even has issues with lead contamination.[208] This is a very sad scenario, and one where very little can be done, but lead is not the only problem in our water supplies.

Several other contaminants should be noted, such as mercury and nitrates. Mercury is not just found in water our fish are swim in, but in our drinking water as well. Mercury toxicity is very harmful to the body and has been linked to numerous health issues such as impaired neurological development,[209] making the presence of mercury a real concern. Nitrates are mostly found in water sources that have been exposed to agricultural contaminants. Then the nitrates convert to nitrites in the body from intestinal bacteria causing compromised red blood cells and their ability to carry oxygen.[210] These contaminants are a growing concern contributing to chronic illness and disease, but we should also be concerned with contaminants that cause acute health issues.

Every year anywhere from 1 to 16 million people fall victim to gastrointestinal illness related to drinking water experiencing symptoms such as nausea, diarrhea, and abdominal cramps.[211] The most vulnerable populations are children, the elderly and individuals with compromised immunity or those undergoing chemotherapy. Even the Environmental Protection Agency recognizes the elderly as truly vulnerable to the effects of contaminated drinking water where diarrhea can often be considered a life-threatening condition.[212]

There are places around the world that do not have near the clean water we do in the United States. We should be grateful we have the water we do relative to underdeveloped areas around the world, but we have to be aware of our own problems as well. Drug-resistant or antibiotic-resistant bacteria make our own water a growing concern. Certain bacteria, when ingested, can cause harm to the human population. When a human being contracts a bacterial infection, an antibiotic is often prescribed. An antibiotic- or drug-resistant bacteria is one has mutated until it is resistant to any kind of drug therapy.

Today, drinking supplies frequently test positive for traces of antibiotic-resistant bacteria.[213] In 2005-2006, the Center for Disease Control reported 20 types of water borne disease outbreaks linked to drinking water, accounting for 612 illnesses and four deaths. These contaminations included bacteria, viruses, and parasites many of which led to upper respiratory illness, gastrointestinal illness and even hepatitis.[214] Many of these outbreaks were further linked to either a water treatment deficiency or untreated water supplies. Another more widespread concern is the use of chlorination, a technique used to purify water. Chlorination actually increases the number of drug-resistant bacteria. Antibiotic resistant bacteria are a huge concern to our health, especially to more vulnerable individuals such as infants, children, pregnant women, the elderly and the immune compromised.[215]

More and more we are beginning to realize our water supplies pose different health risks. Even if you drink only filtered water, you are still exposed to contaminants in your tap water when you bathe and shower in it. Contaminants such as chloroform, tetrachloroethylene, and methyl-t-butyl-ether can be absorbed through the skin while showering or bathing. These contaminants pose a greater risk for pregnant women, children and the elderly.[216] Radon gas, a chemical associated with lung cancer can be released into the air while showering if present in the water.[217]

Water is still the best choice for the body, coming in over caffeinated drinks, sodas, sports drinks, and even fruit juices, but it has to be clean and pure water. If tap water, or many bottled waters are not a good enough choice, what should we drink? Spring water, mineral water, filtered water, distilled water, or reverse osmosis? Spring water is truly only spring water if the label states the source of the spring. Even then you have to decide if the source is acceptable since on occasion you will find the source is a municipal water source. Mineral content varies in spring water as does the contaminants. Drink spring water at your own risk, the same with mineral water. Mineral water usually contains minerals but brands vary in mineral content and contaminants. Trusted brands with detailed labels stating mineral composition and purity can help you choose wisely. Distilled water involves cooking water until it becomes purified steam, and collecting the steam to drink. The upside with distilled water is it is free of all impurities, the down side—it is free of all minerals as well. This may or may not be a problem for the body, research does not agree on whether or not drinking mineral free water is harmful or not.

Right now, with current technologies, carbon block filtration does a decent job of clearing most bacteria, chlorine and chemicals found in tap water while leaving some of the minerals behind. Reverse osmosis is gaining more and more credibility in purifying our tap water. Reverse osmosis will clean everything out of the water, not just bacteria, chlorine and chemicals but also nitrates, fluoride and trace pharmaceuticals that are rumored to be in our tap water.

We cannot take our water for granted, and we have to pay careful consideration to the source and the exposure of our children, our elderly and our immune compromised. We have to realize that, when we turn on a faucet or reach for a case of bottled water, we may not be as risk free as we like to think.

RULE # 15: DRINK CLEAN, PURE WATER.

What you can do right now:

1. Get enough. Adequate hydration is a key piece of the being healthy puzzle. How do you know if you are getting enough? Drink the number of fluid ounces that equals the number of half your body weight in pounds up to but not exceeding one half gallon per day. Example, if you weigh 120 pounds, you need to drink 60 ounces of water every day. If you weigh 250 pounds, you need to drink one half gallon per day and make other necessary changes to bring your weight down. If you weigh more than 250 pounds, do not exceed one gallon of water per day.

2. The real thing. Currently, the closest to perfect water out there is water that has gone through reverse osmosis. Thank goodness there is a way to get pure and clean water. There are plenty of places around the water that do not have access to even moderately clean water.

3. Mineral up. If you are concerned that your drinking water may not have enough minerals, add pink Himalayan sea salt to your meals. Pink Himalayan sea salt is highly alkaline, is full of important minerals, and as mentioned earlier will enhance the flavor of your food.

4. Not in your car. Avoid leaving bottled water in the car. Heat, plastic and water do not make for a winning combination; instead a breeding ground is made for bacteria to multiply. Take it out of the car when you get out.

5. Keep from melting. Many sodas contain high fructose corn syrup, Splenda or aspartame, and phosphoric acid. Phosphoric acid has been known to melt a screwdriver. Imagine what it is doing to your stomach and your intestines?

6. Coffee is not hydration. Caffeine is a diuretic, and this means it will stimulate the body to release more fluid. So, if you drink 8 ounces of a caffeinated drink, you will have to replace the fluid you loose from drinking the caffeine with an additional 8 ounces of water.

7. Dye hair not insides. Human hair will actually take the color of certain kids' drinks when used as temporary hair dye. Apparently it can last on the hair for three weeks or more. If what you are drinking can dye your hair, are you sure you want to pour it into your insides?

8. Children do not need sports drinks. Children today are much more active and participate in many more organized sports. As a result parents believe that sports drinks are a better choice after practice. Many of these drinks are loaded with sugar and food dyes, posing a huge health risk.

9. Bathroom clean. If you are able, a shower and bath filter help reduce the absorption of contaminants through the skin. Especially your children.

PART V

Let's get real about planning.

"To keep the body in good health is a duty, for otherwise
we shall not be able to trim the lamp of wisdom, and
keep our mind strong and clear. Water surrounds
the lotus flower, but does not wet its petals."
—Buddha

CHAPTER SIXTEEN

Simple and not confused.

M Y FATHER LIKED the expression "Keep it simple, stupid." called "KISS" for short. He believed in keeping it very simple when it came to business and marketing strategies, but it is amazing how often you can apply that statement to your entire life and really well to nutrition. After all that we have learned about nutrition in this book so far, I have one more piece of advice for you in this chapter and that is to keep it simple in preparation and in cost. The average meal has over twenty different ingredients especially if your meal contains processed foods and condiments. For example, if you use ready-made bread crumbs in a casserole, the bread crumbs are listed as a single ingredient in your recipe, but the bread crumbs could contain at least a dozen or so ingredients. Certain restaurants are also just as guilty of using a lot of ingredients. Fast food is the worst. A meal from a fast food chain can easily run you in excess of 100 ingredients. Grilled chicken from a certain established fast food chain, (that will go nameless) contains sixty ingredients. The first time I read the list, I thought I had lost count because I could not believe there would be sixty ingredients in a single chicken patty. Try putting into a search engine the fast food chain of your choice, plus the word "ingredients." Take a look at what you are really eating, and then think about it. Really think about it.

It is easy to loose sight of the body's preferred simplicity when it comes to digestion. Since the body is dependent on releasing specific digestive juices based on the kind of food you eat, it makes sense that the simpler your meal, the easier the digestion. A good rule of thumb is to keep meals to seven to twelve ingredients. Seven to twelve ingredients makes for a more easily digested meal while still remaining nutrient dense. Keeping meals to twelve or less ingredients also keeps you from having too many condiments or sauces in one meal. Foods laden with heavy sauces, made with too many condiments, or prepared with refined oils are too complicated for the body to handle cleanly and easily. Baked fish or chicken, steamed veggies, raw fruits and veggies, while keeping sauces or condiments to a minimum can greatly improve digestion.

The biggest obstacles to cooking are our lack of time and energy and the perceived increase in money spent on food. These common complaints keep us from consistently making good choices. If meals were made with a limited amount of ingredients, meal preparation and cooking would go a lot faster. And our bodies would be so much happier. As an added bonus, our grocery bill does not have to be painful.

Here's an example of a simple, 9-ingredient meal that is nutrient dense with red and green foods and at least one raw food, contains protein and is balanced for alkalinity—and is inexpensive and prepares in twenty minutes or less:

» Rice pasta tossed in olive oil with sautéed onion and red bell pepper
» Steamed broccoli

» A raw spinach salad with red onion and goat cheese drizzled with olive oil and lemon juice

When we understand a simpler approach to meal preparation and cooking, then our time in the kitchen is easier and a more pleasant experience.

Another obstacle that deters people from cooking more is the expectation of high grocery bills. Eating real foods begins with buying real foods. Many people avoid making better choices in the grocery store because they believe that healthy food is too expensive. To only a certain degree, they are right. Some health food is more expensive. The idea that *all* healthy food is expensive is a misunderstanding of the big picture. Filet mignon is more expensive than eggs. But good quality eggs are only a few cents more and won't break the grocery budget like steak. Even though cage free eggs are more expensive than conventional eggs, the benefits are worth the extra few cents. We need to understand is that we cannot take care of ourselves cheaply. If we take care of ourselves cheaply, we will get cheap results. The connection between our own health and our budget is that we can pay for our health now or we can pay for it later.

You can make a financial commitment to your health right now. Make the decision to buy better quality food. Making the commitment to better quality food and real ingredients is a much better choice over waiting and seeing what health consequences you will suffer and the medical costs associated with those consequences. You can pay a lot less for your health by being proactive now to prevent chronic illness and disease. Or you can take charge of your current symptoms and improve your health which can save you money in the long run. You have an incredible head start with the rules and strategies in this book, and here are some final tips to help you have everything you need to make a difference in your own health.

Make a 30-day commitment to eating at home. Most of us are working, and many of us have come to believe that we have no time to cook anymore. We have no idea how to cook a simple meal that is not picked up at the drive-thru or served to us at the table in the restaurant, or comes in a box to be heated up in the microwave. Not only do we lack the understanding of how to cook simple meals, but also many of us suffer extreme exhaustion from a poor diet. After a long day at the office, we believe we are too tired to cook, but in actuality we are too exhausted from eating a poor diet that we have no energy or desire to prepare healthy meals. If you made a 30-day commitment to preparing simple meals at home to feel better, at some point during the thirty days you would feel more energy. Once you felt more energy from eating better quality foods, you would feel more motivation to continue preparing healthy meals. When we are unhealthy, we are tired; and when we are tired, we do not make healthy choices. Reverse this cycle. Make healthy meals, feel better and have more energy.

Making healthy meals at home does not mean we have to suddenly become epicures or spend hours in the kitchen. Meals should be simple and easy, and as budget friendly as possible. There are healthy options that take a little bit of preparation in order to be more budget friendly. If we can learn how to desire and prepare simple and healthy meals, then maybe the dollar menu will not have so much financial appeal. With a little help, we can negotiate through the grocery store according to our budget. Statistically it is the lower income neighborhoods that have less access to healthier grocery stores and restaurants and as a result have more nutritionally related health issues,[218] but having access to better grocery stores and restaurants does not always mean we make the best choice. Higher income families will often frequent restaurants more often and, without enough education and understanding, can still suffer nutritionally related illness just like anyone else. Whether you fall into a category of low, middle or high income, it is ultimately your understanding of nutrition that will help you make good choices.

What you have learned in this book can set you apart in the grocery store. Education is the key to health and longevity. Living in a better neighborhood may mean you can shop at better grocery stores more consistently, but there is plenty of damage that can be done to a person's diet no matter where you shop. Eating too much hot dogs and ice cream and avoiding vegetables can cause health issues whether you shop a high end grocery store or a low end grocery store. Expensive ice cream in excess can still be a problem for many people just like the bargain ice cream. Eating vegetables will continue to have tremendous benefits no matter where you grocery shop, even if you cannot afford to buy organic all the time. And eating a bag of cookies over an apple will still have consequences even if the cookie is organic.

The consequences of poor choices exist no matter where you live and shop. We are fortunate enough to live in a country where we have grocery stores, and a lot of them. And now that you have a set of rules and guidelines from this book, your social class does not define what you do about your diet. Being able to afford pastries, bakery items, filet mignon and the finest cuts of meats does not excuse anyone from eating a balanced diet rich in fruits and vegetables. And being on a tight budget does not mean you should shop the dollar menu and deny yourselves the benefits of eating inexpensive quality foods such as eggs, beans, rice, and lots of fruits and vegetables.

Certain healthy food such as grass fed beef is more expensive than grain fed, growth hormone fed beef—but a dozen cage free eggs is less expensive than a pound of beef. Remember you don't need beef or meat in every dinner. Many of us even believe that fruits and vegetables cost too much money in spite of their health benefits.[219] You no longer have to believe the idea that good food is expensive. A bag of apples is approximately the same cost as a large bag of chips, but the bag of apples will last you a lot longer. You can sit down and finish a bag of chips in one or two sittings, but very few of us would sit down and eat 3-4 pounds of apples in one sitting.

Throughout this book, I have given you the information and strategies you need. You now can better understand what healthy eating looks like and may have changed your thinking about what is, and what is not, acceptable to you. By changing your thinking, you have already changed your actions. Remember, you do not have to eat poor quality food in order to survive on a budget; instead, you have to buy the less expensive, high quality food options and know how to prepare them.

Lettuce, apples, peas, carrots, rice, beans, and eggs are some of the most reasonably priced items in a grocery store. Shop outer aisles as much as possible where these fresh items are found. Avoiding prepared mixes and meals that are found in the middle aisles and in the frozen food section will help lower your grocery bill. Avoid food that needs to be microwaved. Avoid packaged snacks. You will be amazed at how you can reduce your grocery bill just by avoiding chips, soda, cookies, candy and keep snacks to fresh fruit, nuts and seeds. On the surface a bag of raw almonds can look like more money than a bag of chips, but a few almonds goes a long way to satisfying the munchies.

Restaurant eating is also another huge expense. Eating out can cost sometimes up to 3-4 times as much as if you prepared that same meal at home. Simple dinners for 4-6 people, when prepared at home, can cost anywhere from $10-$20, but the same type of meal will cost two or three times that amount when purchased at a restaurant. When you reduce the restaurant eating, you will see your actual grocery bill increase. But avoiding a high grocery bill by eating at a restaurant is not really a strategy for lowering your cost of eating. We need to consider our restaurant eating and our grocery bill the same expense, the expense of eating. Then after several months of reducing restaurant eating, see if your total food expense (grocery and restaurant eating) has come down.

Many of you, without realizing it, divide your health expenses into three categories: groceries, medical and eating out/entertainment. Most Americans are spending very little on groceries compared to medical expenses than previous generations. Many people I talk to feel that if they ate better, they would spend more on groceries without even understanding the total cost of eating is reduced. If you are someone who eats out more than prepares meals at home you are spending more money on food than you have to. If you are the chronic restaurant eater, you need a strategy to help you grasp your own nutritional and health finances.

Create a new category called health account. You can keep your subcategories called groceries, medical and eating out as before for tax purposes, but all three now need to be categorized together under the term "health account." You have been learning how much eating affects your health, so at this point you should be ready to actually categorize your groceries as a health expense. Now, examine what you have spent in this area called health account for the past year. Then make the dietary changes suggested in this book for six months, and look at your total health account spending at the end of the six months. And then look again at the end of one year. Your grocery bill may go up, but your eating out should come down significantly. And if you are feeling better, you are likely to have less medical expenses. Then when you look at the combination of groceries, medical and eating out after a year, you will see a lot less in total than you had been spending in previous years. Combining your view of individual expenses into a new single expense called a health account will give you a better perspective on how each of these categories: groceries, eating out and medical all contribute to your health. It will also help you stay committed to your eating as preventative health care and will ultimately save you money by eating higher quality food.

RULE #16: KEEP MEALS SIMPLE IN INGREDIENTS, SIMPLE IN PREPARATION.

What you can do right now:

1. Think 7. Think about your meals in terms of seven to twelve ingredients, and take one meal each week and experiment with simplifying the task, and simplifying the meal and reducing your ingredients. If seven is too limiting, begin with twelve ingredients. If you have been following along, you have already eliminated a lot of processed foods, and you eat more fruits and vegetables. You are now ready to reduce the total number of ingredients at each meal.

2. Ramp up. Start with making the seven to twelve ingredients adjustment at one meal, maybe Monday night dinner. Once you are comfortable with ingredient reduction for that particular dinner take on another day's dinner. After you feel you have mastered a simple fare for the next day, keep going every day until it feels like you have dinner mastered. Then take on lunch.

3. Buy seasonal. Seasonal produce will always be cheaper than out of season, imported produce. Learn what is in season in your area in order to know whether or not you are paying a fair price for produce.

4. Buy fresh or frozen. Frozen vegetables are often less expensive than fresh, and contain as much nutrients. Be careful though, frozen veggies that have been sitting for too long in a freezer will become soggy when prepared and will lose their fresh taste. And if you buy frozen, avoid those with butter and cheese sauces.

5. Buy dried items over canned or boxed mixes. If you are looking for the most inexpensive foods, dried beans and rice are some of the most inexpensive staples. They only take time, not money to be tasty and healthy.

6. Shop the outer aisles. The outer aisles in the grocery store contain the produce, the meat, eggs and other more natural items. You still have to watch since hot dogs and bacon are on the outer aisles, but overall you will find less packaged food on the outer perimeter.

7. Eat eggs over meat if needed. Eggs are an inexpensive and great source of protein and fats.

8. Think again. Next time you have a boxed meal in your hand, see if you can challenge yourself to making it almost as easy but with a lot less burden on your health by making it with less ingredients.

9. Avoid microwave for one week. Make a no microwave zone at your house for one week. This means any meal you had previously microwaved you are now going to make from scratch or prepare something completely different. Make note of how different you should feel after eating a home cooked meal versus a microwaved prefab meal.

10. Make a plan. Plan your dinners for the week in advance, and plan to avoid the restaurants until the weekend. Simple stir-fry, or crock pot meals, soups or meat and veggies can all be prepared simply and easily.

11. Try the meal plan. A one week complimentary meal plan at the end of this book is provided so you can see what this book looks like in action.

12. Commit to your own health with a health account. Combine your groceries, eating out and medical expenses as a single expense called your health. This health account will help you stay committed to nutrition as prevention, and will help you understand a trip to the grocery store may be better for your health and your pocket book in the long run.

Final Words

NOW THAT YOU have completed this book, you can take a stand in favor of a higher quality life through good food. Join the revolution for change, and take a stand against food additives, against imported conventional produce, hormone contaminated meat and dairy, refined cooking oils, refined and processed wheat, and excessive corn and sugar. Take a stand on behalf of organic and local produce, healthy sources of animal protein, healthy fats and oils, eating more alkaline, eating red and green and eating raw at every meal. And watch how you, your spouse and your children evolve on this beautiful journey of eating healthy.

I call you to eat with consciousness, to always remember the connection between what we eat and how we feel, and be a student of your own body. When you connect what you eat with how you feel, your body will speak to you always. You will feel poorly when you stray from the eating naturally. When you stray and feel poorly, allow that moment to be a teaching moment, an opportunity to remind yourself why you no longer eat that way regularly. I have many clients share stories of how eating at a party or eating at a friend's was a revelation to them that day or the next day. I tell them their experience was a great opportunity to understand how disconnected they were before to their eating and how connected and aware they are now. You too, can feel empowered in your eating and your health. Once you have taken responsibility for your eating, you will fully understand how food affects your health and the health of your children.

Our children have suffered long enough from our lack of education about eating. What you have learned in this book is not just for you, but for your children as well. You have a unique opportunity to help your children develop good eating habits. Their health is at stake as well. Think about how many times you go to the doctor or take your children to the doctor, how many times you feel stressed or tired over something your children have said or done, and how often you feel too overwhelmed. By changing your eating and the eating of your children, even if you do so one chapter at a time, or one strategy at a time you will see the difference in your life and the lives of your children. I am well aware that change is not easy, because food is not a small part of our lives. Eating is more than food, eating is about family, and social activities and our traditions. Eating is therefore connected to the quality of our lives, but when we do not prioritize the quality of what we eat, the quality of our lives and our relationships can suffer.

I hope and pray that this book has inspired you toward a greater understanding of the power of what we eat and how it affects our health. From there I hope you have gained some great strategies to help you take the kind of steps you need to take charge of your nutritional health. Hippocrates said "Let food be thy medicine and medicine be thy food." Now you can believe in the wealth of nutrients that are abundant to us if we choose to eat them. And now you know just how to do this. And remember it is not just about your health, but the health of your children and your future generations.

THE RULES FROM *LET'S GET REAL ABOUT EATING*

1. Eat real food.

2. Avoid buying and eating food with high levels of pesticide residue.

3. Know your food, especially the genetically modified stuff.

4. Buy clean animal meat.

5. Change your meat quality, or eat less of it.

6. Choose your dairy products wisely.

7. Eat small fish at least twice a week.

8. Rethink gluten, then reduce or eliminate it from your daily diet.

9. Avoid high fructose corn syrup and genetically modified corn.

10. Avoid artificial sweeteners and reduce sugar consumption.

11. Choose good fats over bad fats, and never go fat free.

12. Eat fruit and veggies daily, but eat twice as many vegetables as you do fruit.

13. Eat the acid alkaline balance of 60/40.

14. Eat red, green and raw at every meal.

15. Drink clean, pure water.

16. Keep meals simple in ingredients, simple in preparation.

Acid Foods	Low	Medium	High
Fruits	Dates Figs	Cranberry	
Veggies		Peas	
Nuts/Seeds		Peanuts Pecans	Walnuts
Oils	Canola Oil Corn Oil Hemp Oil Safflower Oil Sesame Oil Sunflower Oil	Animal Lard	Hydrogenated Oil
Dairy/Eggs	Cow's milk Goat's milk Goat cheese Sheep's milk Yogurt (all) Eggs	Cow's cheese (soft) Sheep's cheese	Cow's cheese (hard)
Meat/Fish		Buffalo Chicken Fish Lamb Oyster Rabbit Scallops Turkey Venison	Beef Lobster Mussels Pork Sausage Shrimp
Grains	Amaranth Hemp Kamut Rice (white and brown) Teff Spelt	Barley Corn Rye Wheat	White flour
Legumes/Beans	Black bean Chick pea Kidney pea Lima bean Navy bean Pinto bean		
Other	Tap water Black tea	Coffee Dark beer	Soda Sugar Hard Liquor Pale Beer

Alkaline Foods	High	Medium	Low
Fruits	Blackberries Cantaloupe Honeydew melon Lemon Pineapple Raspberries Strawberries Tangerine Tropical fruit Watermelon	Apple Apricot Avocado Banana Blueberries Boysenberry Cherries Currants Grapes Grapefruit Pear Peach Orange	Nectarine Plums
Veggies	Asparagus Alfalfa Celery Collard greens Kale Kohlrabi Mustard greens Dandelion greens Onions Pumpkin Rutabaga Wheat grass	Beets Broccoli Cabbage Cauliflower Eggplant Garlic Lettuce Peppers Potatoes Squashes	Brussel sprouts Carrot Chard Cucumber Mushrooms Parsnips Spirulina Sweet potato Sprouts Watercress
Nuts/Seeds	Chestnuts Pumpkin seeds Sprouted seeds		Almonds Brazil nuts Cashews Flax seeds Sesame seeds Sunflower seeds
Oils			Coconut oil Cod liver oil Flax oil Olive oil
Dairy/Eggs			
Meat/Fish			
Grains			Millet Quinoa Oats
Legumes/Beans			Lentils

SAMPLE MEAL PLAN

DAY 1

Breakfast:

Oatmeal-plain (Examples: Quaker's® Old Fashioned or other plain oats)

Fresh blueberries added to oatmeal after cooked

Add almond pieces or almond slices to the bowl of oatmeal

Small glass of orange juice (preferably fresh squeezed and not from concentrate)

Mid-Morning Snack:

Apple (Best choice: Organic, Next best choice: Local)

Lunch:

Sandwich bread (wheat bread made without preservatives such as

Heartland® or Gluten free bread made with non-GMO corn if contains corn)

On the bread add scrambled eggs or homemade egg salad (Options: Spectrum® Organic mayonnaise, or plain yogurt instead of mayonnaise). Add lettuce to sandwich.

Sliced cucumber or zucchini on the side

Sliced strawberries or apple on the side

Or

Chopped Romaine lettuce as a salad base and add the following on top: sliced cucumber, sliced apple, sliced almonds, hardboiled egg, and shredded carrot. Dressing: olive oil and apple cider vinegar.

Afternoon Snack:

Plain organic yogurt (Example: Stoneyfield® Organic or Straus® Organic European style) with fresh fruit added (Example sliced strawberries or blueberries). Drizzle with raw honey (optional)

Or

Cantaloupe and fresh blueberries

Dinner:

Basmati Rice Stir Fry:

Cook the basmati rice and set aside.

Serve with lightly steamed veggies or sautéed lightly in extra virgin olive oil. Vegetable blend example: Red and green bell pepper, onion, zucchini, and broccoli. If steamed, pour olive oil over the vegetables after draining water. Sprinkle with pink Himalayan sea salt and fresh ground pepper. Add slivered almonds or raw cashews to the mixture just before serving.

Salad: Mixed greens with shredded raw carrot. Salad dressing homemade oil and vinegar made with extra virgin olive oil and apple cider vinegar, or olive oil drizzled over the top with fresh squeezed lemon juice.

Day 2

Breakfast:

Quick spinach omelet (Dice spinach small before adding to beaten egg, or sauté spinach first in pan and then add beaten egg over the top) Cook on low with a cover until egg is cooked.

Sliced apple or tomato served on the side

Mid-Morning Snack:

Organic plain yogurt with sliced banana

Or

Banana smoothie with almond milk base (½ c unsweetened almond milk, 1 banana, 2 TB almond or cashew butter, 1 TB raw honey-optional, ½ c ice and blend in blender)

Lunch:

Rice cake (Example: Lundberg® brown rice cakes) with leftover egg salad from yesterday.

Sliced cucumber and Roma tomato salad. Drizzle with olive oil and sprinkle with sea salt. For extra kick sprinkle the cucumber with sesame seeds.

Afternoon Snack:

Celery sticks with almond butter

Or

Organic cottage cheese (Example: Horizon® or Organic Valley®) and sliced pineapple (if using canned pineapple, make sure is in own juices and avoid syrup)

Dinner:

Grilled or baked chicken breast (Best choice: organic, next best choice: range free)

Roasted red potatoes in coconut oil with dried parsley, sea salt and pepper

Steamed frozen peas and carrots

Side salad of chopped Romaine lettuce, sliced cucumber and diced tomato

Day 3

Breakfast:

Poached egg with fresh fruit

Or

Grapefruit and hardboiled egg

Mid–Morning Snack:

Apple

Lunch:

Whole grain tortilla or non–GMO corn tortilla with lettuce, tomato, avocado, and beans.

Or make a quesadilla with tortilla and organic Colby cheese, spinach and sliced tomato.

Afternoon Snack:

Carrot sticks and hummus

Dinner:

Broccoli and Rice:

Cook Basmati or Jasmine rice and set aside.(or can serve this over butternut squash)

Sautee broccoli, onion, mushroom and leeks, diced chicken breast (or ground turkey) in olive oil and season with sea salt and pepper, and serve over rice. (or Garbanzo bean in place of meat for vegetarian night)

Can use a non-GMO tamari soy sauce over the stir-fry for more flavor

Romaine lettuce salad with shredded carrot, diced apple and raisins.

Day 4

Breakfast:

Oatmeal or rice grits (Example: Arrowhead® Rice and Shine hot cereal)

Sliced almonds or diced pecans added to cereal

Blueberries or dried cranberries added to cereal

Morning Snack:

Smoothie (½ c unsweetened almond milk, 1 banana, ½ -1 c frozen berries, ½ c ice)

Lunch:

Cobb Salad:

Diced lettuce and add hardboiled egg (sliced or diced), shredded organic cheese (Colby, cottage or Gouda), diced cucumber and shredded carrot. Extra virgin olive oil and apple cider vinegar salad dressing. (Homemade or Bragg® Healthy Vinaigrette)

Or

Grilled cheese sandwich with side salad of lettuce, cucumber and shredded carrot

Afternoon Snack:

Blend plain organic yogurt with strawberry fruit spread to make into a fruit dip

Slice apples or bananas and dip into fruit dip

Dinner:

Spaghetti or Angel Hair (Examples of Rice pasta: Tinkyada® Pasta Joy, or DeBoles® Rice Pasta) tossed with olive oil after cooked.

Serve with sautéed shrimp (or steamed mussels)

Sautee snow peas, sliced red pepper and broccoli in olive oil. Sprinkle with sea salt and pepper to taste. Toss the vegetables over the top of the shrimp or mussels, or can serve on the side of the pasta with seafood.

Mixed greens salad with goat feta cheese, dried cranberry, sliced red onion and pecans. Mix with extra virgin olive oil and red balsamic vinegar.

Day 5

Breakfast:

French toast (made with cage free eggs and wholesome fresh bread or gluten free bread) served with pure maple syrup and sliced banana or blackberries

Morning Snack

Homemade trail mix of almonds, sunflower seeds, pumpkin seeds, pecans and raisins.

Lunch:

Shrimp bowl:

Leftover shrimp from night before, with shredded raw cabbage

Salsa (watch and avoid brands with sugar) on top

Sliced mango on the side or added to the mixture

Afternoon Snack:

Apple or Pear

Dinner:

Baked sweet potato or homemade sweet potato fries (baked)

Turkey burger (all natural hamburger bun or gluten free or plain)

Peas and onions (sautéed in olive oil)

Green salad with carrots and tomatoes

DAY 6

Breakfast:

Smoothie (½ c almond milk, ½ c pineapple (can be fresh or frozen), 1 banana, ½ c mango chunks, ½ c ice, and blend in blender)

Or

Oatmeal and fresh fruit

Morning Snack:

Avocado

Or

Pineapple (fresh)

Lunch:

Chicken breast or tilapia cooked

Sliced cucumber

Side salad: Sliced strawberries over chopped spinach leaves

Afternoon snack

Organic mozzarella cheese

Small tomatoes

Optional: Chop tomatoes and dice cheese, add chopped basil leaves, extra virgin olive oil and small amount of white balsamic vinegar and toss together as salad

Dinner:

Rice and Tofu Stirfry:

Sautee onion, garbanzo beans, red pepper, spinach and organic tofu. (dice tofu into bite size pieces)

Mix 1 can of tomato paste with 2 cups of plain yogurt in small bowl. Add water to the sauce if too thick. Season as desired and mix the sauce into tofu and vegetable mixture.

Serve over cooked Basmati rice (If adventurous, try quinoa instead of rice. Prepares like rice but with a different flavor)

Side salad of lettuce, sliced oranges, and avocado. Add splash of orange juice to olive oil and white balsamic vinegar and toss over salad.

Day 7

Breakfast:

Rice or oats cold cereal with unsweetened almond milk and blueberries added to cereal

Or

Fruit bowl: sliced banana, strawberries and blueberries

Morning Snack:

Apple with almond butter or roasted almonds

Lunch:

Chicken salad (Diced chicken that is previously cooked), add diced apple, diced celery. Mix with plain yogurt.

Sliced cucumber or zucchini or organic grapes on the side

Afternoon snack

Celery and hummus (or almond butter)

Dinner:

Spaghetti squash (Cut in half and place face down in baking pan with one inch of water on the bottom. Bake at 350 degrees for 30–40 minutes).

Scrape out the squash into bowl. Toss with olive oil and sprinkle with sea salt. Sprinkle with Percino Romano cheese (made from Sheep's milk). Sprinkle with dried parsley

Steamed broccoli served on the side

Salad with lettuce, cucumber, shredded carrot and dried cranberries

BIBLIOGRAPHY AND RESOURCES

Alliance for Bio-Integrity. (2012). Index: Key FDA documents revealing 1) Hazards of genetically engineered foods—and 2) Flaws with how the agency made its policy. Retrieved August 8, 2012 from http://www.biointegrity.org/list.html

Appleton, N. (2009). *Suicide by Sugar: A Startling Look at Our #1 National Addiction.* New York: Square One.

Ballentine, R. (1978) *Diet and Nutrition: A Holistic Approach.* Pennsylvania: The Himalaya International Institute.

Ben, K., Boschiroli, M., Souissi, F., Cherif, N., Benzarti, M., Boukadeda, J., & Hammami, S. (2011). Isolation and molecular characterization of mycobacterium bovis from raw milk in Tunisia. *African Health Sciences*, (S1), S2-S5. PMC3220130

Bernstein, A., Sun, Q., Hu, F., Stampfer, M., Manson, J. & Willett, W. (2010) Major dietary protein sources and risk of coronary heart disease in women. *Circulation*, (122), 876-883. doi:10.1161/circulationaha.109.915165

Black, R., Williams, S., Jones, I., & Goulding, A. (2002). Children who avoid drinking milk have low dietary calcium intake and poor bone health. *American Journal of Clinical Nutrition*, 76(3), 675-680.

Boles, J., Boss, D., Neary, K., Davis, K. & Tess, M. (2008). Growth implants reduced tenderness of steaks from steers and heifers with different genetic potentials for growth and marbling. *JANIM Sci*, 87(1), 269-274. doi:10.2527/jas.2008-1256

Bradbury, J. (2011). Docosahexaenoic Acid (DHA): An acient nutrient for the modern human brain. *Nutrients*, 3(5), 529-554. PMC32557695. doi:10.3390/nu3050529

Braly, J. & Hoggan, R. (2002) *Dangerous Grains*. New York: Penguin Putnam.

Bray, G. (2010). Fructose: pure, white and deadly? Fructose by any other name is a health hazard. *Journal of Diabetes Science and Technology*, 4(4), 1003-1007. PMC290935

Brower, V. (2001). Talking apples and oranges. The EU and the USA continue to struggle over exports of US hormone-treated beef to Europe. *EMBO Reports*, 2(3), 173-174. doi:10.1093/embo-report/kue506

Brown, S & Trivieri, L. (2006). *The Acid Alkaline Food Guide*. New York: Square One.

Burrell, A., Foy, C., & Burns, M., (2011). Applicability of three alternative instruments for food authenticity analysis: GMO identification. *Biotechnology Research International*, 2011:838232. PMC3065168

Bwido, N., & Neumann, C.(2003). The need for animal source food by Kenyan children. *The Journal of Nutrition*. 133(11), 39363S-3940S.

Campbell, T. & Campbell, T (2004). *The China Study: Startling Implications for Diet, Weight Loss and Long Term Health*. Texas: Benbella Books.

Carlisle, T. (1987). FDA's approval of aspartane under scrutiny. *The Globe and Mail Canada*. Retrieved October 2012 , from http://www.wnho.net/fdas_approval_of_aspartane_under_scrutiny.pdf

CDC. (2011). Notes from the field: Yersinia enterocolitica infections associated with pasteurized milk. *Southwestern Pennsylvania*, 60(41), 1428-1428. Retrieved from http://www.cdc.gov

Cisak, E., Wojcik-Fatla, A., Zajac, V., Sroka, J., Buczek, A., & Dukiewicz, J. (2010). Prevalence of tick-borne encephalitis virus (TBEV) in samples of raw milk taken randomly from cows, goats and sheep in Eastern Poland. *Ann Agric EnviroMed*, 17, 283-286. Retrieved from http://www.aaem.pl/pdf/17283.pdf

CNN Health.(2011). More than 1 in 10 in US take antidepressants. Retrieved February 23, 2012 from http://thechart.blogs.cnn.com/2011/10/19/more-than-1-in-10-take-antidepressants.

Colford, J., Helton, J., Wright, C., Arnold, B., Saha, S., Wade, T., Scott, J., & Eisenberg, J. (2009). The Sonoma water evaluation trial; a randomized drinking water intervention trial to reduce gastrointestinal illness in older adults. *American Journal of Public Health*, 99(11), 1988-1995. PMC2759780. doi:10.2105/AJPH.2008.153619

Contento, I. (2011). *Nutrition Education: Linking Research, Theory and Practice*. (2nd Ed). Massachusetts: Jones and Bartlett Publishers.

Cordain, L. (2011). *The Paleo Diet*. (Revised Edition). New Jersey: John Wiley and Sons.

Crook, W. (1986). *The Yeast Connection: A Medical Breakthrough*. New York: Vintage Books.

Curran, L. (2010). EU places warning labels on food containing dyes. *Food Safety News.* Retrieved April 3, 2013 from http://www. foodsafetynews.com/2010/07/eu-places-warning-labels-on-foods-containing-dyes/#.UVzm_6ITLSg

Deriemaeker, P., Aerenhonts, D., Ridder, D., Hebbelinck, M., & Clarys, P. (2011). Health aspects, nutrition and physical characteristics in matched samples of institutionalized vegetarian and non-vegetarian elderly (>65 yrs). *Nutrition & Metabolism*, 8, 37. PMC3135511

Divisi, D., Ditommaso, S., Salvemini, S., Garramone, M., Crisci, R. (2006). Diet and cancer. *ACTA Biomed*, 77, 118-123. Retrieved from www.actabiomedica.it/data/2006/2_2006/divisi.pdf

Duffy, W. (1975). *Sugar Blues.* New York: Grand Central Publishing.

Environmental Working Group. (2011). EWG's 2011 shopper's guide to pesticides in produce. Retrieved November 15, 2011 from http://www.ewg.org/foodnews/list/

EPA. (2012). Agriculture and food supply impacts & adaptation. Retrieved September 1, 2012 from http://www.epa.gov/ climatechange/impacts-adaptation/agriculture.html

EPA (2013). Mercury/Health Effects. Retrieved April 30, 2013 from http://www.epa.gov/hg/effects.htm

Fallon, S. (2001). *Nourishing Traditions: The Cookbook that Challenges Politically Correct Nutrition and the Diet Dictocrats. (*Revised 2nd Edition*)*. Washington D.C.: New Trends Publishing.

Fedoroff, N. (2011) Pusztai's potatoes-Is genetic modification the culprit? Retrieved August 7, 2012, from www.agbioworld. org/biotech-info/articles/biotech-art/pusztai-potatoes.html

Ferguson, L.., Smith, B., & James, B. (2010). Combining nutrition, food science and engineering in developing solutions to inflammatory bowel disease—omega 3 polyunsaturated fatty acids as an example. *Food Function*, 1(1), 60-72. PMID21776456. doi:10.1039/c0fo000057d

Ford, E., Bergmann, M., Kroger, J., Schienkiewits, A., Weiker, C., & Boening, H. (2009). Healthy living is the best revenge. *Arch Intern Med.* 169(15): 1355-1362. doi:10.1001/archinternmed.2009.237

Frahm, A. & Frahm, D. (1992). *A Cancer Battle Plan.* Colorado: Pinion Press.

Fraser, G. (2009). Vegetarian diets: what do we know of their effects on common chronic disease. *The American Journal of Clinical Nutrition,* 89(5), 1607S-1612S. doi:10.3945/ajcn.2009.26736K

Fuhrman, J. (2005). *Disease Proof Your Child: Feeding Kids Right.* New York: St. Martin's Griffin.

Geser, N., Stephan, R., & Hachler, H. (2012). Occurrence and characteristics of extended-spectrum B-lactamase (ESBL) producing Enterobacteriaceae in food producing animals, minced meat and raw milk. *BMC Veterinary Research,* 8(21). PMC3319423. doi:10.1186/1746-6148-8-21

Goodman, R. & Tetteh, A. (2011). Suggested improvements for the allergencity assessment of genetically modified plants used in food. *Current Allergy and Asthma Reports,* 11(4), 317-324. PMC 3130127. doi:10.1007/s11882-011-0195-6

Greenpeace International. (2012). Say no to genetic engineering. *Genetic engineering could be a threat to human and environmental health.* Retrieved August 6, 2012 from http://www.greenpeace.org/international/en/campaigns/agriculture/problem/genetic-engineering/

Haas, E. (1999). *The Staying Healthy Shopper's Guide.* California: Celestial Arts.

Haas, E. & Levin, B. (2006). *Staying Healthy with Nutrition: The Complete Guide to Diet and Nutritional Medicine.* California: Celestial Arts.

Hammad, A., Ahmed, A., Ishida, Y., & Shimamoto, T. (2008). First characterization and emergence of SHV-60 in raw milk of a healthy cow in Japan. *Journal Vet Med Science.* 70(11): 1269-72.

Hetzel, M., Bonfoh, B., Farah, Z., Traore, M....Zinsstag, J. (2004). Diarrhea, vomiting and the role of milk consumption: perceived and identified risk in Bamako (Mali). *Tropical Medicine and International Health*, 9(10), 1132-8.

Hu, Z., Morton, L. & Mahler, R. (2011). Bottled water: United States consumers and their perception of water quality. *International Journal of Environmental Research and Public Health*, 8(2), 565-578. PMC3084479. doi:10.3390/ijerph8028565

Ion, G., Fazio, K., Akinsete, J. & Hardman, E. (2011). Effects of canola and corn oil mimetic on Jurkat cells. *Lipids in Health and Disease*, 10,90. doi:10.1186/1476-511X-10-90

Jacobson, M. (2008). Food dyes should be banned. *BMJ*, 336(7657),1325. PMC2427125. doi:10.1136/bmj.39605.531111.3A

Jaffe, R. (2009). Food Reactivities. *Food and Nutrients in Disease Management.* (pp. 241-259) Florida: CRC Press.

Jaminet, P. & Jaminet, S. (2010). *Perfect Health Diet: Four Steps to Renewed Health, Youthful Vitality and Long Life.* Massachusetts: Ying Yang Press.

Jaynes, W., & Zartman, R. (2011). Aflatoxin toxicity reduction in feed by enhanced binding to surface modified clay additives. *Toxins*, 3(6), 551-565. PMC3202849. doi:10.33901toxins3060531

Jenkins, D., Chiavaroli, L., Wong, J., Kendall, C., Lewis, G....Lamarche, B. (2010) Adding monounsaturated fatty acids to a dietary portfolio of cholesterol lowering foods in hypercholesterolemia. *CMAJ*, 182(18), 1961-1967. PMC3001501. doi: 10.1503/cmaj.092128

Jennings, A., Schwartz, S., Balter, N., Gardner, D., & Witorsch, R. (1990). Effects of oral erythrosine on the pituitary—thyroid axis in rats. *Toxicology Applied Pharmacology*, 103(3), 549-556.

Jonghe, V., Coorevits, A., Hoorde, K., Messens, W., Landschool, A., Vos, P., & Heyndrickx, M. (2011). Influences of storage conditions on the growth of pseudomonas species in refrigerated raw milk. *Applied and Environmental Microbiology*, 77(2), 460-470. PMC 3020527 doi:10.1128/AM.00521-10

Kamer, B., Dolka, E., Pyziak, K., & Blomberg, A. (2011). Food allergy as a cause of constipation in children in the first three years of life-own observations. *Medycyna*, 15(2), 157-161.

Kant, A., Leitzmann, M., Park, Y., Hollenbeck, A., & Schatzkin, A. (2009). Patterns of recommended dietary behaviors predict subsequent risk of mortality in a large cohort of mean and women in the United States. *The Journal of Nutrition*, 139(7), 1374-1380. doi:10-10.3945/

Keith, L. (2009). *The Vegetarian Myth: Food, Justice and Sustainability*. California: Flash Point Press.

Key, T. (2011). Fruit and vegetables and cancer risk. *British Journal of Cancer*, 104(1), 6-11. PMC3039795. doi:10.1038/sj.bjc.6606032

Kiviniemi, M., & Duangdoa, K. (2009). Affective associations mediate the influence of cost benefits on fruit and vegetable consumption. *Appetite*, 52(3), 771-775. PMC2694134. doi:10.1016/j.appetite.2009.02.006

Knowledge Exchange Platform for Responsible Agro-Investment (RAI) (2012). Retrieved August 6, 2012 from gwww.responsibleagroinvestment.org

Kohlstadt, I. (Ed). (2009). *Food and Nutrients in Disease Management*. Florida: CRC Press.

Koutsoumanis, K., Pavlis, A., Nychas, G. & Xanthiakos, K. (2010). Probabilistic model for listeria monocytogens growth during distribution, retail storage, and domestic storage of pasteurized milk. *Applied and Environmental Microbiology*, 76(7), 2181-2191. doi:10.1128/AEM.02430-09

Kuniholm, M., Lesi, O., Mendy, M., Akano, A., Sam, O., Hall, A....Kirk, G. (2008). Aflatoxin exposure and viral hepatitis in the etiology of liver cirrhosis in the Gambia, West Africa. *Environmental Health Perspectives*, 116(11), 1553-1557. PMC 2592277. doi:10.1289/ehp.11661

Lappe, F.M. (1998). *World Hunger: Twelve Myths*. NY: Grove Press.

Lichtenstein, A., Kennedy, E., Barrier, P., Danford, D....Booth, S. (1998). Dietary fat consumption and health. *Nutrition Review*, 56(5Pt2), S3-19, discussion S19-28.

Lipski, E. (2012). *Digestive Wellness: Strengthen the Immune System and Prevent Disease through Healthy Digestion*. (4th Ed) New York: McGraw Hill.

Lobell, D., Schlenker, W., & Costa-Roberts, J. (2012). Climate trends and global crops production since 1980. *Program on Food Security and the Environment Policy Brief*. Retrieved August 7, 2012, from http://fse.standford.edu

Loomis, H. (2007). *Enzymes: The Key to Health, Volume 1*. (3rd Ed) Wisconsin: American Printing Company.

Lopez, S., Bermudez, B., Ortega, A., Varela, L., Pancheo, Y., Villar, J., Abia, R., & Muriana, F. (2011). Effects of meals rich in either monounsaturated or saturated fat on lipid concentrations and on insulin secretion and action in subjects with high fasting triglyceride concentrations. *The American Journal of Clinical Nutrition*, 93(3), 494-499. doi:10.3945/ajcn.110.003251

Margel, D. (2005). *The Nutrient Dense Eating Plan: A Lifetime Eating Guide to Exceptional Foods for Super Health*. California: Basic Health Publications.

Martini, L., & Wood, R. (2009). Milk intake and the risk of Type 2 diabetes mellitus hypertension and prostate cancer. *Arg Bras Endocrinol Metab*, 53(5). Doi:10.1590/s0004-2730200090005000021

Masoodi, T. & Shafi, G. (2010). Analysis of casein alpha S1 & S2 proteins from different mammal species. *Bioinformation*, 4(9), 430-435. PMC 29516535

Mayo Clinic Staff. (2011). *Transfat is double trouble for your heart health.* Retrieved December 11, 2011 from http://www.mayoclinic.com/health/trans-fat/CL00032

Moeller, S., Adamson-Fryhofer, S., Osbahr, A. & Robinowitz, C. (2009) The effects of high fructose corn syrup. *Journal of the American College of Nutrition*, 28(6), 619-626.

Morter, T. (2009). *Your Health…Your Choice…* Florida: Frederick Fell Publishers.

Murray, M., Pizzorno, J. & Pizzorno, L. (2006). *The Encyclopedia of Healing Foods: A User Friendly Guide to the Nutritional Benefits and Medical Properties of Food.* New York: Pocket Books.

Negri, R., DiFeola, M., DiDomenico, S., Scala, M., Artesi, G….Greco, L. (2012). Taste perception and food choices. *Journal of Pediatric Gastroenterology Nutrition*, 54(5), 624-629. doi:10.1097/MPG.0b013e318273308

Ni, X., Wilson, J., Bunton, D., Giro, B., Krakowsky, M., Lee, D….Schmelz, E. (2010). Spatial patterns of aflatoxin levels in relation to ear feeding insect damage in preharvest corn. *Toxins*, 3(7), 920-931. PMC 3202857. doi:10.3390/toxins3070920

Non-GMO Project. (2012). Product Verification: North America's only independent verification of the Noon-GMO products. Retrieved August 7, 2012 http://www.nongmoproject.org/product-verification/

Oates, L. & Cohen, M. (2011). Assessing diet as a modified risk factor for pesticide exposure. *International Journal of Environmental Research and Public Health*, 8(6), 1792-1804. PMC3137997

Olafsdottir, L., Gudjonsson, H., Jonsdottir, H. & Thjodleifsson, B. (2011). National history of heartburn: a 10 year population-based study. *World Journal of Gastroenterology*, 17(5), 639-645.

Oliveira, M. & Osorio, M. (2005). Cow's milk consumption and iron deficiency anemia in children. *Journal of Pediatrics (RioJ)*, 81(5), 361-367.

Oxfam International. (2012). Oxfam International's position on transgenic crops. Retrieved August 6, 2012 from http://www.oxfam.org/en/oxfam-position-transgenic-crops

Pala, V., Krogh, V., Beruno, F., Sieri, S., Grioni, S....Riboli, E. (2009). Meat, eggs, dairy products, and risk of breast cancer in the European Prospective Investigation into Cancer and Nutrition (EPIC) cohort. The American Journal of Clinical Nutrition, 90(3), 602-612. doi:10.3945/ajcn.2008.27173

Pedersen, T., Meilstrup, C., Holstein, B. & Rasmussen, M. (2012). Fruit and vegetable intake is associated with frequency of breakfast, lunch and evening meal: cross sectional study of 11-13 and 15 year olds. *International Journal of Behavioral Nutrition and Physical Activity*, 9(9). PMC331095. doi:10.1186/1479-5868-9-9

Pollan, M. (2009). *Food Rules: An Eater's Manual*. England: Penguin Books.

Pollan, M. (2001). The great yellow hype. *NY Times*. Retrieved August 5, 2012 , from www.nytimes.com/2001/03/04/magazine/04wwln.html

Pitchford, P. (2002). *Healing with Whole Foods: Asian Traditions and Modern Nutrition*. (3rd Edition). California: North Atlantic Books.

Price, W. (2008). *Nutrition and Physical Degeneration*. (9th Ed) California: Price- Pottenger Nutrition Foundation.

Psaltopoulou, T., Kosti, R., Haidopoulos, D., Dimopoulos, M. & Pnangiotakos, D. (2011). Olive oil intake is inversely related to cancer prevalence: a systematic review and a meta-analysis of 13800 patients and 23340 controls in 19 observational studies. *Lipids in Health and Disease*, 10(127). PMC3113199852. doi:10.1186/1476-511x-10-127

Punnen, S., Hardin, J., Cheng, I., Klein, E. & Witte, J. (2011). Impact of meat consumption, preparation, and mutagens on aggressive prostate cancer. *PLoS One*, 6(11), e27711. doi:10.1371/journal.pone.0027711

Pusztai, A. (2012). Genetic engineering-Genetechnology, is it salvation or curse for the 21st century? *Brown Journal*. Retrieved August 7, 2012 , from www.freenetpages.co.uk/hp/a.pusztai/

Renner, R. (2010). Exposure on tap drinking water as an overlooked source of water. *Environmental Health Perspectives*, 118(2), A68-A74. PMC 2831942

Rhodes, J. (1999). Genetically modified foods and the Pusztai affair. *BMJ*, 318(7193):1284.

Richardson, A., Boone-Heinonen, J., Popkin, B. & Gordon-Larsen, P. (2012). Are neighborhood food resources distributed inequitably by income and race in the USA? Epidemiological findings across the urban spectrum. *BMJ*, 2012(2). doi:10.1136/bmjopen-2011-000678

Rippe, J. (2010). The health implications of sucrose, high fructose corn syrup, and fructose: what do we really know? *Journal of Diabetes Science and Technology*, 4(4), 1008-1011. PMC 2909536

Rodrigo, L. (2006). Celiac disease. *World Journal Gastroenterology*, 12(41), 6585-6593.

Ronald, P. (2011). Plant genetics, sustainable agriculture and global food security. *Genetics,* 188(1), 11-20. doi:10.1534/genetics.111.128553

Ryan-Harshman, M. & Alsoori, W. (2007). Diet and colorectal cancer. *Canadian Family Physician,* 53(11):1913-1920. PMC2231486

Science Daily. (2007). Culinary shocker: cooking can preserve, boost nutrient content of vegetables. Retrieved November 19, 2012 from http://www.sciencedaily.com/releases/2007/12/071224125524.htm

Shibko, S. (1992). Memorandum from Dr. Samuel I. Shibko to Dr. James Maryanski, FDA Biotechnology Coordinator. *Subject: "Revision of toxicology section of the statement of policy: foods derived from genetically modified plants".* Retrieved August 8, 2012 from www.biointegrity/FDAdocs/03/view1.html

Smith, J. (2007). *Genetic Roulette: The Documented Health Risks of Genetically Engineered Food.* Iowa: Yes! Books.

Soechtig, S. & Lindsey, J. (Directors). (2009). *Tapped* [Documentary]. United States. Atlas Films.

Spiroux de Vendomois, J., Celleir, D., Velot, C., Clair, E., Mesnage, R., & Sealini, G. (2010). Debate on GMO's health rises after statistical findings in regulatory tests. *International Journal of Biological Sciences,* 6(6), 590-598.

The Hunger Project. (2012). Enpowering women and men to end their own hunger. Retrieved August 6, 2012 from www.thp.org

Tiffin, R. & Salois, M. (2012). Inequalities in diet and nutrition. *Proceedings of the Nutrition Society,* 71(1), 105-111. doi:10.1017/S0029665111003284

Valcke, M. & Krishnan, K. (2010). An assessment of the interindividual variability of internal dosimetry during multi-route exposure to drinking water contaminants. *International Journal of Environmental Research and Public Health,* 7(11), 4002-4022. PMC 2996221. doi:10.3390/ijerph7114002

Wang, T., Zhang, E., Chen, X., Li, L. & Liang, X.(2010). Identification of seed proteins associated with resistance to preharvested aflatoxin contamination in peanut (arachis hypo gaea L). *BMC Plant Biology,* 10(267). PMC3095339. doi:10.1186/1471-2229-10-267

Waserman, S., & Watson, W. (2011). Food allergy. *Allergy, Asthma & Clinical Immunology,* 7(Suppl 1), S7. PMC3245440

Weiss, B. (2012). Synthetic food colors and the neurobehavioral hazards: the view from environmental health research. *Environmental Health Perspective,* 120(1), 1-5. PMC 3261946. doi 10.1289/ehp.1103827

Xi, C., Zhang, Y., Marrs, C., Ye, W., Simon, C., Foxman, B. & Nriagu, J. (2009). Prevalence of antibiotic resistance in drinking water treatment and distribution systems. *Applied and Environmental Microbiology,* 75(17), 5714-5718. PMC2737933. doi:10.1128/AEM.00382-09

Yam, D., Eliraz, A. & Berry, E. (1996). Diet and disease-the Israeli paradox: possible dangers of a high omega-6 polyunsaturated fatty acid diet. *Is J Med Sci,* 32(11), 1134-1143.

Yang, O. (2010). Gain weight by "going diet" artificial sweeteners and the neurobiology of sugar cravings. *Yale Journal of Biology and Medicine,* 83(2), 101-108, PMC 2892-765

Yoder, J., Roberts, V., Crawn, G., Hill, V., Hick, L....Roy, S. (2008). Surveillance for waterborne disease and outbreaks associated with drinking water and water not intended for drinking-United States, 2005-2006. *MMWR Surveill Summ,* 54(40), 1105, and 57(9), 39-62.

Zender, R., Bachard, A. & Reif, J. (2001). Exposure to tap water during pregnancy. *Journal of Exposure Science and Environmental Epidemiology,* 11, 224-230. doi:10.1038/sj.jea.7500163

ENDNOTES

1. Ford, E., Bergmann, M., Kroger, J., Schienkiewits, A., Weiker, C., & Boening, H. (2009). Healthy living is the best revenge. *Arch Intern Med.* 169(15): 1355-1362. doi:10.1001/archinternmed.2009.237

2. Fuhrman, J. (2005). *Disease Proof Your Child: Feeding Kids Right.* New York: St. Martin's Griffin. p 72

3. Frahm, A. & Frahm, D. (1992). *A Cancer Battle Plan.* Colorado: Pinion Press. p 115

4. Rippe, J. (2010). The health implications of sucrose, high fructose corn syrup, and fructose: what do we really know? *Journal of Diabetes Science and Technology*, 4(4), 1008-1011. PMC 2909536

5. Lipski, E. (2012). *Digestive Wellness: Strengthen the Immune System and Prevent Disease through Healthy Digestion.* (4th Ed) New York: McGraw Hill. p 89

6. Pollan, M. (2009). *Food Rules: An Eater's Manual.* England: Penguin Books. p 5

7. Contento, I. (2011). *Nutrition Education: Linking Research, Theory and Practice.* (2nd Ed). Massachusetts: Jones and Bartlett Publishers. p 4

8. Haas, E. (1999). *The Staying Healthy Shopper's Guide.* California: Celestial Arts. p 13

9.   Jennings, A., Schwartz, S., Balter, N., Gardner, D., & Witorsch, R. (1990). Effects of oral erythrosine on the pituitary—thyroid axis in rats. *Toxicology Applied Pharmacology*, 103(3), 549-556.

10.   Weiss, B. (2012). Synthetic food colors and the neurobehavioral hazards: the view from environmental health research. *Environmental Health Perspective*, 120(1), 1-5. PMC 3261946. doi 10.1289/ehp.1103827

11.   Ibid

12.   Jacobson, M. (2008). Food dyes should be banned. *BMJ*, 336(7657),1325. PMC2427125

13.   Curran, L. (2010). EU places warning labels on food containing dyes. *Food Safety News*. Retrieved April 3, 2013 from http://www.foodsafetynews.com/2010/07/eu-places-warning-labels-on-foods-containing-dyes/#.UVzm_6ITLSg

14.   Jacobson, M. (2008). Food dyes should be banned. *BMJ*, 336(7657),1325. PMC2427125

15.   Olafsdottir, L., Gudjonsson, H., Jonsdottir, H. & Thjodleifsson, B. (2011). National history of heartburn: a 10 year population-based study. *World Journal of Gastroenterology,* 17(5), 639-645.

16.   Ronald, P. (2011). Plant genetics, sustainable agriculture and global food security. *Genetics,* 188(1), 11-20. doi:10.1534/genetics.111.128553

17.   Haas, E. (1999). *The Staying Healthy Shopper's Guide*. California: Celestial Arts. p 29

18.   Ibid. p 18-21

19.   Oates, L. & Cohen, M. (2011). Assessing diet as a modified risk factor for pesticide exposure. *International Journal of Environmental Research and Public Health*, 8(6), 1792-1804. PMC3137997

20.   Haas, E. (1999). *The Staying Healthy Shopper's Guide*. California: Celestial Arts. p 30

21.   Ibid, p 22-29

22.   Ibid, p24

23.   Smith, J. (2007). *Genetic Roulette: The Documented Health Risks of Genetically Engineered Food*. Iowa: Yes! Books. p 1

24.   Pollan, M. (2001). The great yellow hype. *NY Times*. Retrieved August 5, 2012 , from www.nytimes.com/2001/03/04/magazine/04wwln.html

25. Greenpeace International. (2012). Say no to genetic engineering. *Genetic engineering could be a treat to human and environmental health.* Retrieved August 6, 2012 from http://www.greenpeace.org/international/en/campaigns/agriculture/problem/genetic-engineering/

26. Ronald, P. (2011). Plant genetics, sustainable agriculture and global food security. *Genetics,* 188(1), 11-20. doi:10.1534/genetics.111.128553

27. The Hunger Project. (2012). Enpowering women and men to end their own hunger. Retrieved August 6, 2012 from www.thp.org

28. EPA. (2012). Agriculture and food supply impacts & adaptation. Retrieved August 6, 2012 from http://www.epa.gov/climatechange/impacts-adaptation/agriculture.html

29. Lobell, D., Schlenker, W., & Costa-Roberts, J. (2012). Climate trends and global crops production since 1980. *Program on Food Security and the Environment Policy Brief.* Retrieved August 7, 2012 from http://fse.standford.edu

30. Lappe, F.M. (1998). *World Hunger: Twelve Myths.* NY: Grove Press. p 9

31. Knowledge Exchange Platform for Responsible Agro-Investment (RAI) (2012). Retrieved August 6, 2012 from gwww.responsibleagroinvestment.org

32. Oxfam International. (2012). Oxfam International's position on transgenic crops. Retrieved August 6, 2012 from http://www.oxfam.org/en/oxfam-position-transgenic-crops

33. Smith, J. (2007). *Genetic Roulette: The Documented Health Risks of Genetically Engineered Food.* Iowa: Yes! Books. p 240

34. Ibid

35. Ronald, P. (2011). Plant genetics, sustainable agriculture and global food security. *Genetics,* 188(1), 11-20. doi:10.1534/genetics.111.128553

36. Lobell, D., Schlenker, W., & Costa-Roberts, J. (2012). Climate trends and global crops production since 1980. *Program on Food Security and the Environment Policy Brief.* Retrieved August 7, 2012 from http://fse.standford.edu

37. Spiroux de Vendomois, J., Celleir, D., Velot, C., Clair, E., Mesnage, R., & Sealini, G. (2010). Debate on GMO's health rises after statistical findings in regulatory tests. *International Journal of Biological Sciences,* 6(6), 590-598.

38. Greenpeace International. (2012). Say no to genetic engineering. *Genetic engineering could be a threat to human and environmental health.* Retrieved August 6, 2012 from http://www.greenpeace.org/international/en/campaigns/agriculture/problem/genetic-engineering/

39. NON-GMO Project. (2012). Product Verification: North America's only independent verification of the Noon-GMO products. Retrieved August 7, 2012 http://www.nongmoproject.org/product-verification/

40. Goodman, R. & Tetteh, A. (2011). Suggested improvements for the allergencity assessment of genetically modified plants used in food. *Current Allergy and Asthma Reports*, 11(4), 317-324. PMC 3130127. doi:10.1007/s11882-011-0195-6

41. Smith, J. (2007). *Genetic Roulette: The Documented Health Risks of Genetically Engineered Food*. Iowa: Yes! Books. p 143-171

42. Ibid, p 59

43. Ibid, p 7

44. Spiroux de Vendomois, J., Celleir, D., Velot, C., Clair, E., Mesnage, R., & Sealini, G. (2010). Debate on GMO's health rises after statistical findings in regulatory tests. *International Journal of Biological Sciences*, 6(6), 590-598.

45. Smith, J. (2007). *Genetic Roulette: The Documented Health Risks of Genetically Engineered Food*. Iowa: Yes! Books. p 27

46. Pusztai, A. (2012). Genetic engineering-Genetechnology, is it salvation or curse for the 21st century? *Brown Journal*. Retrieved August 7, 2012 , from www.freenetpages.co.uk/hp/a.pusztai/

47. Fedoroff, N. (2011) Pusztai's potatoes-Is genetic modification the culprit? Retrieved August 7, 2012, from www.agbioworld.org/biotech-info/articles/biotech-art/pusztai-potatoes.html

48. Smith, J. (2007). *Genetic Roulette: The Documented Health Risks of Genetically Engineered Food*. Iowa: Yes! Books. p 22

49. Alliance for Bio-Integrity. (2012). Index: Key FDA documents revealing 1) Hazards of genetically engineered foods—and 2) Flaws with how the agency made its policy. Retrieved August 8, 2012 from http://www.biointegrity.org/list.html

50. Shibko, S. (1992). Memorandum from Dr. Samuel I. Shibko to Dr. James Maryanski, FDA Biotechnology Coordinator. Subject: "Revision of toxicology section of the statement of policy: foods derived from genetically modified plants". Retrieved August 8, 2012 from www.biointegrity/FDAdocs/03/view1.html

51. Brower, V. (2001). Talking apples and oranges. The EU and the USA continue to struggle over exports of US hormone-treated beef to Europe. *EMBO Reports*, 2(3), 173-174. doi:10.1093/embo-report/kue506

52. Fuhrman, J. (2005). *Disease Proof Your Child: Feeding Kids Right.* New York: St. Martin's Griffin. p 89-90

53. Brower, V. (2001). Talking apples and oranges. The EU and the USA continue to struggle over exports of US hormone-treated beef to Europe. *EMBO Reports,* 2(3), 173-174. doi:10.1093/embo-report/kue506

54. Ibid

55. Ibid

56. Ibid

57. Ibid

58. Cordain, L. (2011). *The Paleo Diet.* (Revised Edition). New Jersey: John Wiley and Sons. p 52

59. Ibid, p 80

60. Ibid, p 217

61. Fallon, S. (2001). *Nourishing Traditions: The Cookbook that Challenges Politically Correct Nutrition and the Diet Dictocrats.* (Revised 2nd Edition). Washington D.C.: New Trends Publishing. p 27

62. Price, W. (2008). *Nutrition and Physical Degeneration.* (9th Ed) California: Price-Pottenger Nutrition Foundation.

63. Fallon, S. (2001). *Nourishing Traditions: The Cookbook that Challenges Politically Correct Nutrition and the Diet Dictocrats.* (Revised 2nd Edition). Washington D.C.: New Trends Publishing. p 27

64. Campbell, T. & Campbell, T (2004). *The China Study: Startling Implications for Diet, Weight Loss and Long Term Health.* Texas: Benbella Books. p 6

65. Pitchford, P. (2002). *Healing with Whole Foods: Asian Traditions and Modern Nutrition.* (3rd Edition). California: North Atlantic Books. p 29

66. Cordain, L. (2011). *The Paleo Diet.* (Revised Edition). New Jersey: John Wiley and Sons. p 11

67. Murray, M., Pizzorno, J. & Pizzorno, L. (2006). *The Encyclopedia of Healing Foods: A User Friendly Guide to the Nutritional Benefits and Medical Properties of Food.* New York: Pocket Books. p 13

68. Ibid, p 13

69. Ryan-Harshman, M. & Alsoori, W. (2007). Diet and colorectal cancer. *Canadian Family Physician,* 53(11):1913-1920. PMC2231486

70. Punnen, S., Hardin, J., Cheng, I., Klein, E. & Witte, J. (2011). Impact of meat consumption, preparation, and mutagens on aggressive prostate cancer. *PLoS One*, 6(11), e27711. doi:10.1371/journal.pone.0027711

71. Divisi, D., Ditommaso, S., Salvemini, S., Garramone, M., Crisci, R. (2006). Diet and cancer. *ACTA Biomed*, 77, 118-123. Retrieved from www. actabiomedica.it/data/2006/2_2006/divisi.pdf

72. Fallon, S. (2001). *Nourishing Traditions: The Cookbook that Challenges Politically Correct Nutrition and the Diet Dictocrats.* (Revised 2nd Edition). Washington D.C.: New Trends Publishing. p 29

73. Ford, E., Bergmann, M., Kroger, J., Schienkiewits, A., Weiker, C., & Boening, H. (2009). Healthy living is the best revenge. *Arch Intern Med.* 169(15): 1355-1362. doi:10.1001/archinternmed.2009.237

74. Jaminet, P. & Jaminet, S. (2010). *Perfect Health Diet: Four Steps to Renewed Health, Youthful Vitality and Long Life.* Massachusetts: Ying Yang Press. p 9

75. Fuhrman, J. (2005). *Disease Proof Your Child: Feeding Kids Right.* New York: St. Martin's Griffin. p 68

76. Fallon, S. (2001). *Nourishing Traditions: The Cookbook that Challenges Politically Correct Nutrition and the Diet Dictocrats.* (Revised 2nd Edition). Washington D.C.: New Trends Publishing. p 35

77. Ibid, p 33

78. Fuhrman, J. (2005). *Disease Proof Your Child: Feeding Kids Right.* New York: St. Martin's Griffin. p 33

79. Martini, L., & Wood, R. (2009). Milk intake and the risk of Type 2 diabetes mellitus hypertension and prostate cancer. *Arg Bras Endocrinol Metab*, 53(5). Doi:10.1590/s0004-2730200090005000021

80. Fallon, S. (2001). *Nourishing Traditions: The Cookbook that Challenges Politically Correct Nutrition and the Diet Dictocrats.* (Revised 2nd Edition). Washington D.C.: New Trends Publishing. p 34-35

81. Fuhrman, J. (2005). *Disease Proof Your Child: Feeding Kids Right.* New York: St. Martin's Griffin. p 69

82. Fallon, S. (2001). *Nourishing Traditions: The Cookbook that Challenges Politically Correct Nutrition and the Diet Dictocrats.* (Revised 2nd Edition). Washington D.C.: New Trends Publishing. p 34

83. Koutsoumanis, K., Pavlis, A., Nychas, G. & Xanthiakos, K. (2010). Probabilistic model for listeria monocytogens growth during distribution, retail storage, and domestic storage of pasteurized milk. *Applied and Environmental Microbiology*, 76(7), 2181-2191. doi:10.1128/AEM.02430-09

84. Hammad, A., Ahmed, A., Ishida, Y., & Shimamoto, T. (2008). First characterization and emergence of SHV-60 in raw milk of a healthy cow in Japan. *Journal Vet Med Science*. 70(11): 1269-72.

85. Ben, K., Boschiroli, M., Souissi, F., Cherif, N., Benzarti, M., Boukadeda, J., & Hammami, S. (2011). Isolation and molecular characterization of mycobacterium bovis from raw milk in Tunisia. *African Health Sciences*, (S1), S2-S5. PMC3220130

86. Hetzel, M., Bonfoh, B., Farah, Z., Traore, M....Zinsstag, J. (2004). Diarrhea, vomiting and the role of milk consumption: perceived and identified risk in Bamako (Mali). *Tropical Medicine and International Health*, 9(10), 1132-8.

87. Cisak, E., Wojcik-Fatla, A., Zajac, V., Sroka, J., Buczek, A., & Dukiewicz, J. (2010). Prevalence of tick-borne encephalitis virus (TBEV) in samples of raw milk taken randomly from cows, goats and sheep in Eastern Poland. *Ann Agric EnviroMed*, 17, 283-286. Retrieved from http://www.aaem.pl/pdf/17283.pdf

88. Jonghe, V., Coorevits, A., Hoorde, K., Messens, W., Landschool, A., Vos, P., & Heyndrickx, M. (2011). Influences of storage conditions on the growth of pseudomonas species in refrigerated raw milk. *Applied and Environmental Microbiology*, 77(2), 460-470. PMC 3020527 doi:10.1128/AM.00521-10

89. Fuhrman, J. (2005). *Disease Proof Your Child: Feeding Kids Right*. New York: St. Martin's Griffin. p 68

90. Masoodi, T. & Shafi, G. (2010). Analysis of casein alpha S1 & S2 proteins from different mammal species. *Bioinformation*, 4(9), 430-435. PMC 29516535

91. Kamer, B., Dolka, E., Pyziak, K., & Blomberg, A. (2011). Food allergy as a cause of constipation in children in the first three years of life-own observations. *Medycyna*, 15(2), 157-161.

92. Masoodi, T. & Shafi, G. (2010). Analysis of casein alpha S1 & S2 proteins from different mammal species. *Bioinformation*, 4(9), 430-435. PMC 29516535

93. Ibid

94. Ibid

95. Bradbury, J. (2011). Docosahexaenoic Acid (DHA): An acient nutrient for the modern human brain. *Nutrients*, 3(5), 529-554. PMC32557695

96. Murray, M., Pizzorno, J. & Pizzorno, L. (2006). *The Encyclopedia of Healing Foods: A User Friendly Guide to the Nutritional Benefits and Medical Properties of Food.* New York: Pocket Books. p 575-576

97. Ibid, p 574

98. Ibid, p 580-581

99. Ibid, p 580

100. Ibid, p 591

101. Braly, J. & Hoggan, R. (2002) *Dangerous Grains.* New York: Penguin Putnam.p xii

102. Ibid

103. Jaffe, R. (2009). Food Reactivities. *Food and Nutrients in Disease Management.* (pp. 241-259) Florida: CRC Press. p 241-259

104. Ballentine, R. (1978) *Diet and Nutrition: A Holistic Approach.* Pennsylvania: The Himalaya International Institute. p 66-75

105. Ibid, p 66-75

106. Ibid, p 66-75

107. Margel, D. (2005). *The Nutrient Dense Eating Plan: A Lifetime Eating Guide to Exceptional Foods for Super Health.* California: Basic Health Publications.

108. Cordain, L. (2011). *The Paleo Diet.* (Revised Edition). New Jersey: John Wiley and Sons. p 55-59

109. Ibid, p 93

110. Ibid, p 96

111. Moeller, S., Adamson-Fryhofer, S., Osbahr, A. & Robinowitz, C. (2009) The effects of high fructose corn syrup. *Journal of the American College of Nutrition*, 28(6), 619-626.

112. Ibid

113. Ibid

114. Ibid

115. Appleton, N. (2009). *Suicide by Sugar: A Startling Look at Our #1 National Addiction.* New York: Square One. p 62-63

116. Rippe, J. (2010). The health implications of sucrose, high fructose corn syrup, and fructose: what do we really know? *Journal of Diabetes Science and Technology*, 4(4), 1008-1011. PMC 2909536

117. Yang, O. (2010). Gain weight by "going diet" artificial sweeteners and the neurobiology of sugar cravings. *Yale Journal of Biology and Medicine*, 83(2), 101-108, PMC 2892-765

118. Yang, O. (2010). Gain weight by "going diet" artificial sweeteners and the neurobiology of sugar cravings. *Yale Journal of Biology and Medicine*, 83(2), 101-108, PMC 2892-765

119. Appleton, N. (2009). *Suicide by Sugar: A Startling Look at Our #1 National Addiction.* New York: Square One. p 60

120. Ion, G., Fazio, K., Akinsete, J. & Hardman, E. (2011). Effects of canola and corn oil mimetic on Jurkat cells. *Lipids in Health and Disease*, 10,90. doi:10.1186/1476-511X-10-90

121. Ibid

122. Jaminet, P. & Jaminet, S. (2010). *Perfect Health Diet: Four Steps to Renewed Health, Youthful Vitality and Long Life.* Massachusetts: Ying Yang Press. p 57-61

123. Ibid, p 61

124. Ni, X., Wilson, J., Bunton, D., Giro, B., Krakowsky, M., ...Lee, D. (2010). Spatial patterns of aflatoxin levels in relation to ear feeding insect damage in preharvest corn. *Toxins*, 3(7), 920-931. PMC 3202857. doi:10.3390/toxins3070920

125. Jaynes, W., & Zartman, R. (2011). Aflatoxin toxicity reduction in feed by enhanced binding to surface modified clay additives. *Toxins*, 3(6), 551-565. PMC3202849. doi:10.33901toxins3060531

126. Ni, X., Wilson, J., Bunton, D., Giro, B., Krakowsky, M., ...Lee, D. (2010). Spatial patterns of aflatoxin levels in relation to ear feeding insect damage in preharvest corn. *Toxins*, 3(7), 920-931. PMC 3202857. doi:10.3390/toxins3070920

127. Jaynes, W., & Zartman, R. (2011). Aflatoxin toxicity reduction in feed by enhanced binding to surface modified clay additives. *Toxins*, 3(6), 551-565. PMC3202849. doi:10.33901toxins3060531

128. Duffy, W. (1975). *Sugar Blues.* New York: Grand Central Publishing. p 30

129. Appleton, N. (2009). *Suicide by Sugar: A Startling Look at Our #1 National Addiction.* New York: Square One. p 8

130. Ibid, p 57

131. Ibid, p 59

132. Ibid, p 56

133. Ibid, p 82

134. Ibid, p 83

135. Ibid, 85

136. Ibid, p 13-19

137. CNN Health.(2011). More than 1 in 10 in US take antidepressants. Retrieved February 23, 2012 from http://thechart.blogs.cnn.com/2011/10/19/more-than-1-in-10-take-antidepressants.

138. Ibid

139. Appleton, N. (2009). *Suicide by Sugar: A Startling Look at Our #1 National Addiction.* New York: Square One. p 14

140. Rippe, J. (2010). The health implications of sucrose, high fructose corn syrup, and fructose: what do we really know? *Journal of Diabetes Science and Technology,* 4(4), 1008-1011. PMC 2909536

141. Yang, O. (2010). Gain weight by "going diet" artificial sweeteners and the neurobiology of sugar cravings. *Yale Journal of Biology and Medicine,* 83(2), 101-108, PMC 2892-765

142. Ibid

143. Carlisle, T. (1987). FDA's approval of aspartane under scrutiny. *The Globe and Mail Canada.* Retrieved October 2012 , from http://www.wnho.net/fdas_approval_of_aspartane_under_scrutiny.pdf

144. Ibid

145. Cordain, L. (2011). *The Paleo Diet.* (Revised Edition). New Jersey: John Wiley and Sons. p 13

146. Jaminet, P. & Jaminet, S. (2010). *Perfect Health Diet: Four Steps to Renewed Health, Youthful Vitality and Long Life.* Massachusetts: Ying Yang Press. p 65

147. Cordain, L. (2011). *The Paleo Diet.* (Revised Edition). New Jersey: John Wiley and Sons. p 51

148. Mayo Clinic Staff. (2011). *Transfat is double trouble for your heart health.* Retrieved December 11, 2011 from http://www.mayoclinic.com/health/trans-fat/CL00032

149. Pitchford, P. (2002). *Healing with Whole Foods: Asian Traditions and Modern Nutrition.* (3rd Edition). California: North Atlantic Books. p 180-181

150. Jenkins, D., Chiavaroli, L., Wong, J., Kendall, C., ...Lewis, G. (2010) Adding monounsaturated fatty acids to a dietary portfolio of cholesterol lowering foods in hypercholesterolemia. *CMAJ*, 182(18), 1961-1967. PMC3001501. doi: 10.1503/cmaj.092128

151. Ibid

152. Lopez, S., Bermudez, B., Ortega, A., Varela, L., Pancheo, Y., Villar, J., Abia, R., & Muriana, F. (2011). Effects of meals rich in either monounsaturated or saturated fat on lipid concentrations and on insulin secretion and action in subjects with high fasting triglyceride concentrations. *The American Journal of Clinical Nutrition*, 93(3), 494-499. doi:10.3945/ajcn.110.003251

153. Psaltopoulou, T., Kosti, R., Haidopoulos, D., Dimopoulos, M. & Pnangiotakos, D. (2011). Olive oil intake is inversely related to cancer prevalence: a systematic review and a meta-analysis of 13800 patients and 23340 controls in 19 observational studies. *Lipids in Health and Disease*, 10(127). PMC3113199852. doi:10.1186/1476-511x-10-127

154. Fraser, G. (2009). Vegetarian diets: what do we know of their effects on common chronic disease. *The American Journal of Clinical Nutrition*, 89(5), 1607S-1612S. doi:10.3945/ajcn.2009.26736K

155. Science Daily. (2007). Culinary shocker: cooking can preserve, boost nutrient content of vegetables. Retrieved November 19, 2012 from http://www.sciencedaily.com/releases/2007/12/071224125524.htm

156. Murray, M., Pizzorno, J. & Pizzorno, L. (2006). *The Encyclopedia of Healing Foods: A User Friendly Guide to the Nutritional Benefits and Medical Properties of Food.* New York: Pocket Books. p 47

157. Pitchford, P. (2002). *Healing with Whole Foods: Asian Traditions and Modern Nutrition.* (3rd Edition). California: North Atlantic Books. p 537

158. Murray, M., Pizzorno, J. & Pizzorno, L. (2006). *The Encyclopedia of Healing Foods: A User Friendly Guide to the Nutritional Benefits and Medical Properties of Food.* New York: Pocket Books. p 50

159. Pitchford, P. (2002). *Healing with Whole Foods: Asian Traditions and Modern Nutrition.* (3rd Edition). California: North Atlantic Books. p 537

160. Murray, M., Pizzorno, J. & Pizzorno, L. (2006). *The Encyclopedia of Healing Foods:* A User Friendly Guide to the Nutritional Benefits and Medical Properties of Food. New York: Pocket Books. p 62

161. Pitchford, P. (2002). *Healing with Whole Foods: Asian Traditions and Modern Nutrition*. (3rd Edition). California: North Atlantic Books. p 539

162. Murray, M., Pizzorno, J. & Pizzorno, L. (2006). *The Encyclopedia of Healing Foods: A User Friendly Guide to the Nutritional Benefits and Medical Properties of Food*. New York: Pocket Books. p 68

163. Ibid, p 72

164. Ibid, p 72

165. Pitchford, P. (2002). *Healing with Whole Foods: Asian Traditions and Modern Nutrition*. (3rd Edition). California: North Atlantic Books. p 538

166. Ibid, p 538

167. Ibid, p 540

168. Murray, M., Pizzorno, J. & Pizzorno, L. (2006). *The Encyclopedia of Healing Foods: A User Friendly Guide to the Nutritional Benefits and Medical Properties of Food*. New York: Pocket Books. p 83

169. Ibid, p 83

170. Ibid, 129

171. Pitchford, P. (2002). *Healing with Whole Foods: Asian Traditions and Modern Nutrition*. (3rd Edition). California: North Atlantic Books. p 549

172. Murray, M., Pizzorno, J. & Pizzorno, L. (2006). *The Encyclopedia of Healing Foods: A User Friendly Guide to the Nutritional Benefits and Medical Properties of Food*. New York: Pocket Books. p 148-149

173. Ibid, p 154

174. Ibid, p 154

175. Ibid, p 158

176. Ibid, p 158

177. Pitchford, P. (2002). *Healing with Whole Foods: Asian Traditions and Modern Nutrition*. (3rd Edition). California: North Atlantic Books. p 550

178. Kiviniemi, M., & Duangdoa, K. (2009). Affective associations mediate the influence of cost benefits on fruit and vegetable consumption. *Appetite*, 52(3), 771-775. PMC2694134. doi:10.1016/j.appetite.2009.02.006

179. Murray, M., Pizzorno, J. & Pizzorno, L. (2006). *The Encyclopedia of Healing Foods: A User Friendly Guide to the Nutritional Benefits and Medical Properties of Food*. New York: Pocket Books.

180. Jaminet, P. & Jaminet, S. (2010). *Perfect Health Diet: Four Steps to Renewed Health, Youthful Vitality and Long Life*. Massachusetts: Ying Yang Press.

181. Pitchford, P. (2002). *Healing with Whole Foods: Asian Traditions and Modern Nutrition.* (3rd Edition). California: North Atlantic Books. p 263

182. Jaminet, P. & Jaminet, S. (2010). *Perfect Health Diet: Four Steps to Renewed Health, Youthful Vitality and Long Life.* Massachusetts: Ying Yang Press.

183. Ryan-Harshman, M. & Alsoori, W. (2007). Diet and colorectal cancer. *Canadian Family Physician,* 53(11):1913-1920. PMC2231486

184. Murray, M., Pizzorno, J. & Pizzorno, L. (2006). *The Encyclopedia of Healing Foods: A User Friendly Guide to the Nutritional Benefits and Medical Properties of Food.* New York: Pocket Books. p 176

185. Environmental Working Group. (2011). EWG's 2011 shopper's guide to pesticides in produce. Retrieved November 15, 2011 from http://www.ewg.org/foodnews/list/

186. Murray, M., Pizzorno, J. & Pizzorno, L. (2006). *The Encyclopedia of Healing Foods: A User Friendly Guide to the Nutritional Benefits and Medical Properties of Food.* New York: Pocket Books.

187. Cordain, L. (2011). *The Paleo Diet.* (Revised Edition). New Jersey: John Wiley and Sons. p 19

188. Ibid, p 19 and 54

189. Ibid, p 18

190. Frahm, A. & Frahm, D. (1992). *A Cancer Battle Plan.* Colorado: Pinion Press.

191. Brown, S & Trivieri, L. (2006). *The Acid Alkaline Food Guide.* New York: Square One.

192. Loomis, H. (2007). *Enzymes: The Key to Health, Volume 1.* (3rd Ed) Wisconsin: American Printing Company. p 89-91

193. Ibid, p 111

194. Ibid, p 110-115

195. Ibid, p 115

196. Ibid, p 91

197. Haas, E. & Levin, B. (2006). *Staying Healthy with Nutrition: The Complete Guide to Diet and Nutritional Medicine.* California: Celestial Arts. p 14

198. Hu, Z., Morton, L. & Mahler, R. (2011). Bottled water: United States consumers and their perception of water quality. *International Journal of Environmental Research and Public Health,* 8(2), 565-578. PMC3084479. doi:10.3390/ijerph8028565

199. Ibid

200. Soechtig, S. & Lindsey, J. (Directors). (2009). *Tapped* [Documentary]. United States. Atlas Films.

201. Haas, E. & Levin, B. (2006). *Staying Healthy with Nutrition: The Complete Guide to Diet and Nutritional Medicine.* California: Celestial Arts. p 17

202. Ibid, p 18

203. Ibid

204. Ibid

205. Ibid

206. Renner, R. (2010). Exposure on tap drinking water as an overlooked source of water. *Environmental Health Perspectives,* 118(2), A68-A74. PMC 2831942

207. Ibid

208. Ibid

209. EPA (2013). Mercury/Health Effects. Retrieved April 30, 2013 from http://www.epa.gov/hg/effects.htm

210. Haas, E. & Levin, B. (2006). *Staying Healthy with Nutrition: The Complete Guide to Diet and Nutritional Medicine.* California: Celestial Arts. p 19

211. Colford, J., Helton, J., Wright, C., Arnold, B., Saha, S., Wade, T., Scott, J., & Eisenberg, J. (2009). The Sonoma water evaluation trial; a randomized drinking water intervention trial to reduce gastrointestinal illness in older adults. *American Journal of Public Health,* 99(11), 1988-1995. PMC2759780. doi:10.2105/AJPH.2008.153619

212. Ibid

213. Xi, C., Zhang, Y., Marrs, C., Ye, W., Simon, C., Foxman, B. & Nriagu, J. (2009). Prevalence of antibiotic resistance in drinking water treatment and distribution systems. *Applied and Environmental Microbiology,* 75(17), 5714-5718. PMC2737933. doi:10.1128/AEM.00382-09

214. Yoder, J., Roberts, V., Crawn, G., Hill, V., Hick, L....Roy, S. (2008). Surveillance for waterborne disease and outbreaks associated with drinking water and water not intended for drinking-United States, 2005-2006. *MMWR Surveill Summ,* 54(40), 1105, and 57(9), 39-62

215. Xi, C., Zhang, Y., Marrs, C., Ye, W., Simon, C., Foxman, B. & Nriagu, J. (2009). Prevalence of antibiotic resistance in drinking water treatment and distribution systems. *Applied and Environmental Microbiology,* 75(17), 5714-5718. PMC2737933. doi:10.1128/AEM.00382-09

216. Valcke, M. & Krishnan, K. (2010). An assessment of the interindividual variability of internal dosimetry during multi-route exposure to drinking water contaminants. *International Journal of Environmental Research and Public Health*, 7(11), 4002-4022. PMC 2996221. doi:10.3390/ijerph7114002

217. Haas, E. & Levin, B. (2006). *Staying Healthy with Nutrition: The Complete Guide to Diet and Nutritional Medicine*. California: Celestial Arts. p 19

218. Richardson, A., Boone-Heinonen, J., Popkin, B. & Gordon-Larsen, P. (2012). Are neighborhood food resources distributed inequitably by income and race in the USA? Epidemiological findings across the urban spectrum. *BMJ*, 2012(2). doi:10.1136/bmjopen-2011-000678

219. Kiviniemi, M., & Duangdoa, K. (2009). Affective associations mediate the influence of cost benefits on fruit and vegetable consumption. *Appetite*, 52(3), 771-775. PMC2694134. doi:10.1016/j.appetite.2009.02.006

About the Author

Laura Kopec, ND, MHNE, CNC received her Doctorate in Traditional Naturopathy from Trinity School of Natural Health, a Master of Arts from the University of Arizona, a Master of Science in Health and Nutrition Education from Hawthorn University, and a Nutritional Counseling Certificate from Trinity School of Natural Health. Laura has a unique background in communications, presentation, education, nutrition, whole body wellness and natural living. Laura is a consultant, educator, speaker and author. She has a consulting practice in Plano, Texas where she lives with her husband and three children. She is available for consultations in person or by phone; and she is available for speaking engagements. She is also the founder of Kopec Naturals natural skincare products. You can find out more about her and her work at www.kopecnaturals.com

INDEX

A

Acid alkaline | 110, 113–115, 148, 162, 187
Aflatoxin | 78, 166, 168, 169, 173, 183
Almonds | 9, 49, 53, 54, 72, 73, 88, 107, 114, 122, 124, 140, 151–153, 155–158
Amino acid | 29, 33, 38, 42, 49
Animal rennet | 52, 53, 54
Antibiotic resistant | 129
Antioxidants | 100, 103, 105, 118
Appetite control | 77, 85
Apple | 7, 9, 30, 83, 103–107, 113, 114, 116, 118, 121, 124, 139, 140, 151–156, 158, 162, 178, 179
Arthritis | 58, 69, 84, 91, 93, 100, 126
Artificial colors | 4, 6, 10
Artificial ingredient | 3, 4, 5, 10, 42, 55, 107
Aspartame | 55, 86–88, 131

Autoimmune disease | 67, 68, 69, 93

B

Banana | 7, 9, 104, 116, 153, 155–158
Bottled water | 126, 129, 130, 131, 166, 187
Bottom feeders | 60, 61
Brain tumor | 39, 85
Breast cancer | 30, 170
British Foods Standard Agency | 6
Broccoli | 7, 44, 100, 101, 106, 115, 118, 122, 123, 136, 152, 154, 156, 159

C

Cabbage | 49, 101, 106, 156
Calcium | 49, 53, 54, 58, 61, 68, 71, 73, 101, 102, 105, 111, 112, 162
California Department of Agriculture | 13

Cancer | xix, xx, 12, 21, 30, 32, 33, 38–42, 49, 52, 58, 60, 67, 76–78, 84, 85, 92, 100–103, 105, 106, 112, 129, 164, 165, 167, 169–172, 175, 179, 180, 185–187

Canola oil | 24, 77, 91, 94

Carbon block filtration | 130

Carrot | 7, 9, 49, 72, 100–102, 108, 113, 122–124, 140, 152, 154, 155, 157, 159

Celiac | xix, 67, 69, 70, 93, 171

Center for Disease Control | 50, 128

Cheese | 31, 48, 52, 52–54, 55, 66, 106, 137, 142, 153–157, 159

Chlorination | 127, 129

Coconut oil | 78, 90, 92–95, 100, 111, 115, 154

Colby cheese | 54, 154

Colon cancer | 40, 52, 101

Constipation | 52, 112, 119, 120, 125, 126, 167, 181

Corn | xx, 5, 18, 19, 21, 23, 24, 44, 65, 66, 73, 75–78, 79, 80, 83, 85, 87, 94, 100, 104, 131, 145, 147, 152, 154, 166, 169, 171, 175, 182–184

Corn oil | 76–79, 94, 166, 183

D

Dairy | 30, 34, 35, 42, 44, 47, 49–53, 54, 55, 66, 92, 99, 113, 115, 145, 147, 170

Diabetes | xix, xx, 41, 48, 49, 52, 69, 76, 77, 85, 91, 103, 105, 126, 162, 169, 171, 175, 180, 183, 184

Digestive enzymes | 119, 121

DNA | 18, 21

Dopamine | 84

Dr. Feingold | 5

Dr. Weston Price | 33, 37, 50

E

Environmental Protection Agency (EPA) | 12, 19, 30, 126

Environmental Working Group (EWG) | 13, 105

Enzymes | 48, 52, 53, 105, 118–120, 121, 168, 187

European Union | 6, 31

Extra virgin olive oil | 92, 94, 95, 100, 115, 123, 152, 155–157

F

Farmer's market | 9, 15, 24

Fast food | 29, 39, 42, 94, 104, 135, 136

Fat soluble vitamins | 89

Fermentation | 54

Food additives | 145

Food Advisory Committee | 5

Food and Drug Administration | 5, 22, 23, 25, 31, 85, 161, 163, 172, 178, 184

Food dye | 5, 6, 10, 55, 60, 131, 166, 176

Food enzymes | 119, 120

Food sensitivities | xviii, 67, 68

Fruit | 5, 6, 8, 9, 12–16, 33, 66, 69, 70, 72, 99, 100, 103–105, 106–108, 111, 114, 116, 119–122, 124, 126, 129, 136, 139–141, 148, 152, 154, 155, 157, 158, 167, 170, 186, 189

G

Genetically modified food | 17–23, 18, 25, 171

Genetically modified organism | 17, 18, 19, 20, 21, 22, 23, 24, 25, 75,

79, 80, 152, 154, 155, 162, 169, 172, 177, 178

Gluten | 65, 65–70, 71–73, 147, 152, 156, 157

Gluten sensitivity | 67, 70

Goat milk | 53, 55

Gouda cheese | 54, 155

Grass fed | 32, 34, 41, 43, 54, 92, 122, 139

Greenpeace | 18, 21, 59, 61, 165, 177

Growing population | 20

H

Health account | 141, 143

Heartburn | 71, 170, 176

Heirloom garden | 24

High cholesterol | 32, 76, 84, 114

High fructose corn syrup | xx, 5, 65, 66, 75–78, 79, 83, 85, 87, 104, 131, 147, 169, 171, 175, 183, 184

Hormones in dairy | 49

Hormones in meat | 31

Hot dogs | 39, 41–43, 107, 139, 142

Hydrogenated oil | 90, 91, 93

I

Illegal pesticide | 13, 15

Infertility | 12, 21, 41

Inflammation | xvii, xix, 32, 77, 91, 93, 100, 102

Ingredient | 3, 4–10, 12, 24, 39, 42, 52, 55, 66, 75–77, 79, 82, 86–88, 105, 107, 110, 115, 120, 123, 135–137, 141, 142, 148

K

Klebsiella pneumonia | 50

L

Lactase | 48, 54

Lactose intolerant | 48

Lead contamination | 127

Leukemia | 12, 39

M

Magnesium | 49, 101, 102, 105, 111, 112, 120

Marine Conservation Society | 61

Mayo Clinic | 90, 169, 184

Meal plan | 151

Meat quality | 43, 147

Mercury | 58, 59, 61, 127, 128, 164, 188

Metabolic acidosis | 110

Metabolic enzymes | 119, 121

Metabolic syndrome | 76

Metabolism | 66, 68, 91, 92, 164

Michael Pollan | 4, 18, 170, 175, 176

Microwave | 40, 43, 138, 143

Monounsaturated | 90, 91, 92, 166, 168, 185

Mosanto | 22

Mozzarella | 54, 157

Mycotoxin | 78

N

National Primary Drinking Water Standards | 126

Nitrates | 39, 43, 128, 130

Non-GMO verified | 79

O

Obesity | xix, 7, 31, 76, 77, 83, 84, 114

Omega 3 | 32, 57, 58, 60, 61, 91–93, 95, 164

Omega 6 | 32, 77, 91–93

Organic | xi, 11, 14–16, 15, 23, 24, 34, 41, 44, 50, 53–55, 59–61, 80, 83, 92, 94, 95, 105, 107, 113, 115, 139, 145, 151–155, 157, 158

Osteoporosis | 47, 91, 111

P

Paleo Diet | 32, 37, 38, 68, 72, 90, 111, 163, 179, 182, 184, 187

Papaya | 21, 23

Partially hydrogenated oil | 90, 91, 93

Pasteurization | 49, 50, 105

Pesticides | 11–13, 14–16, 53, 54, 58, 105, 111, 113, 127, 164, 187

Pink Himalayan sea salt | 94, 108, 131, 152

Polyunsaturated | 77, 90–94, 104, 164, 173

Prostate cancer | 12, 30, 40, 42, 49, 101, 169, 171, 180

Pusztai's research | 22, 164, 171, 178

R

Range free | 34, 153

Raw food diet | 121, 122

Raw milk | 50, 51, 161, 163, 165–167, 181

Real food | xi, 3, 6–11, 39, 71, 82, 118, 137, 147

Red dye #3 | 5

Refined carbohydrates | 65, 66, 67, 69, 72, 107, 111, 120

Reverse osmosis | 129, 130

S

Salmon | 23, 29, 58–61

Salmonella | 50

Serotonin | 84

Sodium benzoate | 5

Soy | 8, 24, 41, 54, 155

Spinach | 29, 100, 102, 103, 106, 108, 118, 122, 137, 153, 154, 157, 158

Sports drinks | 86, 129, 131

Spring water | 129

Stomach acid | 102

Sugar | 4, 23, 24, 33, 44, 54, 55, 65, 66, 75–78, 81–84, 85–88, 102–105, 107, 108, 115, 131, 145, 147, 156, 161, 164, 173, 183–185

Sweeteners | 55, 76, 77, 81, 82, 85–88, 147, 173, 183, 184

T

Tap water | 108, 126, 127, 129, 130, 173

The China Study | 38, 162, 179

Thyroid | 5, 12, 167, 176

Transfat | 65, 90, 93, 169, 184

Triglycerides | 77, 93

Turmeric | 59, 61

U

US Geological Survey | 127

V

Vegan | 38, 40, 40–42, 44, 114

Vegetable rennet | 52, 53, 54

Vegetables | 6, 15, 16, 33, 41, 45, 66, 69, 70, 72, 79, 80, 92, 94, 99–103, 104, 106–108, 111, 113–115, 120, 122, 124, 126, 139, 141, 142, 148, 152, 156, 167, 172, 185

Vegetarian | 37, 38, 40–42, 41, 44, 99, 109, 114, 154, 164, 165, 167, 185

Vitamin B12 | 29, 33, 42, 59

W

Weston Price Foundation | 37, 50
White flour | 39, 65–68, 70–72, 107, 115
World Health Organization | xix, 38
World hunger | 19, 168, 177

Y

Yersinia enterocolitica | 50, 163
Yogurt | 9, 48, 52, 54, 55, 86, 152, 153, 155, 158

Printed in the United States
By Bookmasters